SCHIZOPHRENIA

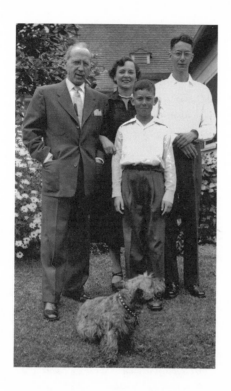

SCHIZOPHRENIA

A Brother Finds Answers in Biological Science

Ronald Chase

The Johns Hopkins University Press
Baltimore

© 2013 The Johns Hopkins University Press
All rights reserved. Published 2013
Printed in the United States of America on acid-free paper
9 8 7 6 5 4 3 2 1

The Johns Hopkins University Press
2715 North Charles Street
Baltimore, Maryland 21218-4363
www.press.jhu.edu

Chase, Ronald.
    Schizophrenia : a brother finds answers in biological science / Ronald Chase.
        pages cm
    Includes index.
    ISBN 978-1-4214-1090-6 (hardcover : alk. paper) — ISBN 978-1-4214-1091-3
(pbk. : alk. paper) — ISBN 978-1-4214-1092-0 (electronic) — ISBN 1-4214-1090-7
(hardcover : alk. paper) — ISBN 1-4214-1091-5 (pbk. : alk. paper) — ISBN
1-4214-1092-3 (electronic)
    1. Schizophrenia.   2. Schizophrenia in adolescence.   3. Schizophrenics—
Family relationships—United States.   4. Neuropsychiatry.   I. Title.
    RC514.C463 2014
    616.89'8—dc23   2013001717

A catalog record for this book is available from the British Library.

Special discounts are available for bulk purchases of this book. For more information,
please contact Special Sales at 410-516-6936 or specialsales@press.jhu.edu.

The Johns Hopkins University Press uses environmentally friendly book
materials, including recycled text paper that is composed of at least 30 percent
post-consumer waste, whenever possible.

For Zanna and Aaron

They too are siblings

Contents

Acknowledgments

I thank Irving Gottesman, Ph.D., Andrew Shaner, M.D., and Rajiv Tandon, M.D., who provided me with valuable suggestions after reading an early version of the manuscript. Many thanks also to Jacqueline Wehmueller of the Johns Hopkins University Press for her enthusiasm, good judgment, and superb editing. My wife, Dorothy Chase, encouraged me and, in so many other ways, kept me going.

SCHIZOPHRENIA

Prologue

Schizophrenia is an illness that frightens and fascinates, but few people know much about it. Yes, it is generally known that schizophrenia is a serious mental illness. And, yes, people know that occasionally a person who commits a violent act can escape criminal penalties if he or she is proved to have schizophrenia. But the symptoms of the disease, who gets it, and its fundamental nature remain blurred, even in the minds of people who have known its victims. Medical science has itself been slow to understand the disease. The history of **psychiatry*** is filled with wild speculations, false hypotheses, and ill-conceived treatments, which have led people to entertain fuzzy and sometimes romantic ideas, for example, that schizophrenia is caused by bad mothering or God's will, that it is simply an extreme form of social deviance, or even that it is a *good* thing because it comes with creativity.

After centuries of ignorance, those who seek to learn the facts are now confronted with an entirely different problem: the overwhelming number of scientific and medical publications. In 1958, the year in which my own brother, Jim, became ill, 474 journal articles were published on the subject of schizophrenia. Thereafter, the pace of publication steadily quickened until, by 2012, the annual total was 5,766 articles. There are now more than 100,000 English-language articles directly related to schizophrenia (dating from 1930 to 2013), most of which are readily available to academics and researchers on the Web.[1] Despite the great

*The glossary at the end of the book contains explanations for technical and unfamiliar words. Items that appear in the glossary are highlighted when they first appear in the text.

quantity of research, the science of schizophrenia remains unsettled. Making sense of the staggering amount of information means sifting through reams of material to separate the solid research from the shoddy research, recognizing false leads, and reconciling contradictions. With an average of around 100 new publications appearing every week, keeping up to date can be daunting.

There is another difficulty in learning about schizophrenia: only those who suffer from it truly know what it is like to have the disease. With most other illnesses, patients can describe their symptoms in detail, and they can report on the subjective feelings that accompany them. Schizophrenia robs its victims of the insights and the verbal skills required for such descriptions. Also, **stigma** silences those who might otherwise speak out.

Because of my dual roles of loving brother and professional biologist, I have been motivated to write a book that gives a more complete view of schizophrenia, one that presents in alternating chapters both a personal story and an objective account. The objective chapters that cover the medical and scientific facts of schizophrenia bear titles in the form of questions. These are the questions that I struggled with over the course of my brother's life and that I needed to answer for myself. I assume that many readers will have been seeking answers to the same, or similar, questions.

The chapters that tell the story of my brother's illness follow an irregular chronology that omits large chunks of time. In part this is because I lived far away from Jim during most of my adult life and saw him only intermittently. But also, I decided it would be better to look more closely at a few pivotal events rather than attempt a narrative that would include every twist and turn of his illness. Because I was not in constant contact with my brother, I witnessed only a few of the episodes of **psychosis** during which he suffered from **paranoiac delusions**. Whereas bizarre or dramatic behaviors are often the focus of biographical accounts of schizophrenia, in my brother's case, and I suspect in most other cases, it is the crippled navigation of everyday life that is more representative. Thus, I hope that the biographical chapters in this book will reveal both the nature of the illness and the character of the person who was my brother.

I cannot claim that Jim represented a typical case of schizophrenia, for the simple reason that I do not believe there exists *any* typical case. Nor was his a *stereo*typical case, by which I mean a case involving horrible acts of violence, as the popular (mis)conception would have it. As I will explain, schizophrenia is a poorly defined disease that takes many different forms. Jim was essentially a quiet and unobtrusive person. Most of the time, except during the occasional relapse, his medications worked well in controlling the worst manifestations of his disease, the so-called **positive symptoms** of schizophrenia, which in Jim's case included delusions, **disorganized speech**, and auditory **hallucinations**. They failed, however, to relieve his so-called **negative symptoms**, which included social withdrawal, the absence of motivation, and depression. Whether Jim's symptoms and the progression of his illness match those of any other persons with the same illness is less important than the fact that all people with schizophrenia suffer tragically. It pains me to know that Jim never had a serious relationship with a woman, had no children, was unable to continue his promising career, and so much more.

Schizophrenia is a disease that affects not only the person who has the disease but also that person's family. Thus, my brother's story is also my own story, and my mother's and father's (I have no other siblings). Again, the particulars of my family's experiences will differ from those of other families, but the burden of guilt and the anguish of unanswered questions will be familiar to everyone whose loved ones have suffered from schizophrenia.

The science of schizophrenia currently comprises a myriad of facts and a few highly contested hypotheses. The pursuit of definitive answers is neither just beginning nor close to ending; rather, it is at an exciting stage somewhere in between. Scientists are drawn to research in schizophrenia because they see it as a big puzzle, and scientists love to solve puzzles. Moreover, many scientists, including myself, believe that by studying schizophrenia we may learn a considerable amount about how the normal brain works. Novel approaches and new methodologies are continuously being brought to bear on the issues raised by schizophrenia. I hope to convey some of this excitement in my book.

I must enter a caveat in regard to the scientific and medical facts related here. Inevitably, as with any such summary of a complex subject, mine is biased by the author's point of view. My account reflects a special interest in the disciplines of **neuroscience**, **genetics**, and **epidemiology** and a preference for rigorous, usually quantitative, investigations. I have highlighted the research that in my opinion is the most significant and the most representative of current knowledge, but as I have mentioned, the literature is vast, and opinions differ. Moreover, because new publications keep appearing at an astonishingly high rate, it is impossible to be entirely up to date.

When my brother had his first psychotic episode, in 1958, America was in the midst of a postwar economic boom. Although the times were generally good for most people in Los Angeles, they were far from okay for people with schizophrenia. People who had schizophrenia were often treated with electroconvulsive shock, and, if that treatment was unsuccessful, they were confined to dreary state-run hospitals. A group of intellectuals, forming an antipsychiatry movement, had gained a loyal following by arguing that mental illness was nothing but a social myth. Neuroscience was in its infancy, antipsychotic drugs had only just entered North America, and the concept of community care was still unborn in North America. I, as a teenager, was struggling to find answers to the many questions I had concerning my brother.

This book is about Jim and his disease, but it is appropriate for me to explain why I have written it, and to do so, I need to recount some of my own life. My entire adult life has been shadowed by my brother's illness and the need to understand what happened to him but not to me. At university, I studied the disciplines that seemed to offer answers. In and out of classrooms, I immersed myself in psychology, **psychoanalysis**, and existential philosophy. I remember reading a heavy tome written by Jean-Paul Sartre called *Being and Nothingness* (in translation), and another volume entitled *Existential Psychiatry*. I also read the centerpiece of the antipsychiatry movement, a book with the audacious title, *The Myth of Mental Illness*. These and other books left me confounded with all the competing ideas about the causes of, and the treatments for, schizophrenia. After graduation, I attempted to stifle my fascination with psychiatry, and to remove myself from the pain of Jim's illness, by enrolling in a law school far away from my home. However, with the questions still unanswered, the distress continued. What had happened to Jim, and why *him*? What, exactly, is mental illness?

Slowly, I came to realize that mental illness is not in the mind, but rather in the brain. I cannot say exactly how this happened, but I know that this insight marked a major turning point in my life. The first big decision that I took as a consequence of this insight was to leave Harvard Law School. I spent the next year working as a bookseller, reading, and thinking. Then, having decided to look at psychiatry from a new perspective, I took a job as a research assistant at the Massachusetts Mental Health Center. With my eyes finally opened to the possibilities of science, I enrolled in a graduate program that promised to teach me about the brain. From that point onward, I have looked upon schizophrenia as a scientific problem, one that can be solved by examining evidence and testing hypotheses. Schizophrenia is a disease rooted in human biology. Through research, we will find ways to treat it effectively and perhaps even prevent it. I have found peace of mind in this approach, and I hope that the reader will too.

Let me explain why I do not call anyone a "schizophrenic" in this book. People who are knowledgeable about mental health issues recoil when they hear this expression. Rightly so, I believe, because no one should be defined by his or her illness. People with schizophrenia have attributes in addition to their illnesses, things such as personalities, talents, and interests. Rather than saying that a person *is* schizophrenic, I speak of persons *who have* schizophrenia. It is a small linguistic difference but a meaningful one for those affected by the disease. Moreover, studies have shown that the use of the label "schizophrenic" contributes to the creation of stigma.

1

Innocence on the Road to Los Angeles

As in most families who later have to contend with schizophrenia, we saw no early signs of the trouble that lay ahead. Looking back at my childhood, which corresponded to the beginning of Jim's teen years, I recall only conventional pleasures. When schizophrenia did eventually come crashing down upon us, it arrived with all the weight of a tidal wave. The pivotal event left us in no doubt that everything in our lives was about to change.

In 1958, Jim was a 25-year-old graduate student at the University of California, Los Angeles (UCLA). He was living off-campus when his thinking became horribly disturbed, his fears became irrational, and his contact with reality became dangerously thin. In short, he experienced a psychotic breakdown, which is the way that schizophrenia usually begins.

It was late on a weekday afternoon. I was passing time in my room, reading a borrowed Hardy Boys book, when the phone rang. I ignored the ring, but someone else picked up the phone in another room. Shortly afterward I heard Mom shout, "*Joe, he has a gun!*"

I reached for the phone extension above my bed.

"Where are you?" Mom was asking Jim.

"Where do you think I am?" Jim answered in an angry tone. "I'm at my apartment."

He spoke in a loud and sometimes sputtering voice. "There's a girl here," he declared. "It's her fault. She's making me do it. Bitch!"

"*What* is her fault, Jimmy? *What* is she making you do?"

"Oh no Mother, you know perfectly well what she is up to. Why do you pretend that you don't know?"

"Jimmy dear, please, I'm not pretending. Calm down and tell me what is happening over there."

"I'll tell you what's happening," Jim said. He was talking fast now, slurring his words and slipping into incoherence. "She won't admit that it's her fault. Damn the bitch! She can go to hell! I'll shoot her first, *then* she can go to hell. That's the way to stop this stuff. I can't stand it any longer. I'm going to shoot her and then shoot myself."

Jim was born in Chicago in the middle of the Great Depression. As a baby, he was as cute and cuddly as a child can be. Writing in his diary on the first anniversary of Jim's birth, Dad described him as "probably the sweetest little guy that ever lived. He can smile and laugh and play to make one see heaven on earth right in that little fellow. What is more lovely than to behold Jimmy's mother holding her son in her arms, playing with him and loving him?" In his youth, Jim was strikingly handsome, with clear blue eyes, dark wavy hair, and the unmistakable appearance of intelligence. His mild manners and exceptional study habits set him apart from most of the other boys at school.

By the end of the Second World War, the economy was booming again, and American families were on the move. Dad had managed to put aside some money and was considering a change too. One day in the spring of 1948, he announced to Jim and me that the family would be moving to Los Angeles. By this time, Jim was 14 years old and already six feet tall. He was lanky and awkward and wore horned rim glasses. It was obvious that he preferred reading books to rough-and-tumble play.

Jim was seven years older than I. We were brothers from the start, but we only became friends when we shared the backseat of Dad's Chevrolet on our trip to California. Dad drove and Mom sat beside him. Our itinerary followed the fabled U.S. Route 66 from Chicago to Los Angeles. For me, at age 7, it was a grand adventure and great fun. I enjoyed the sights and the experiences, but most of all, I enjoyed being with my family. All those warm memories, however, are wrapped in the hindsight knowledge that the trip marked a passage from our family's happy

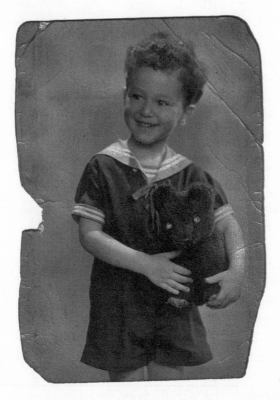

Jim in 1937, 3½ years old

years in Chicago to our troubled years in Los Angeles. Much later, when I asked Dad whether it was Jim's illness that had prompted the move, he unhesitatingly replied no and added that it was simply a matter of getting away from the harsh Chicago winters. There was nothing to hint at the trouble that lay not 2,448 miles ahead but rather 10 years in the future.

On the way to Los Angeles, Jim sat beside me reading books, presumably novels. Although I myself read an occasional comic book, I did not read nearly as much as he did—neither then nor later. I occupied myself mostly by working mechanical puzzles. There was one where you moved small tiles so that they would appear in numerical sequence. I also had a set of paired wires that were tangled together like a knot; the object of the puzzle was to untangle the knot. Meanwhile, Dad was always at the wheel, driving attentively and with pleasure, for he had been fond of automobiles ever since his father bought an early Ford Model T. It would not be correct to say, however, that Dad's attention was 100 percent riveted on the road. He was continuously distracted with his tobacco pipes. The only time a pipe was not stuck in his mouth was when he had consumed all of its tobacco.

Despite Mom's protests, Dad kept one hand on the wheel and used the other to empty and clean the exhausted pipe. He put away the cleaned pipe and picked up another of his favorites, which he immediately began to load with his favorite brand of tobacco, Revelation. Again using his free hand, he dipped the pipe into the pouch of tobacco, filled the bowl with tobacco, packed it with his fingers, and finished by tamping and trimming the loose shreds with a special tool. Next, he struck a match and, with the pipe in his mouth, he drew the flame onto the tobacco. A cloud of sweet smelling smoke soon filled the car. The pipe bowl glowed with hot tobacco embers. Mom protested wearily, "Joe, can't you live without that damned pipe for even a few minutes? You're making a mess in here and you're going to start a fire!" Reluctantly, Dad reached for a small, metallic screen, and he clamped it in place on top of the burning mass. He took a couple of deep puffs to make sure that the combustion was unimpeded, then relaxed. "How about a game of 20 questions?" he asked.

"Ronnie, it's your turn to think of something." I thought real hard for a few minutes then announced that I was ready, "Okay, it's *animal*. Mom, it's your turn to start."

"Let's see . . . Is it a person?"

"Yes, it is."

Jim, "Is the person alive?"

"No."

Dad, "Someone we know personally?"

"No."

Mom again, "Male?"

"Yes."

Jim, "Musician?"

"No."

Dad, "Novelist?"

"No."

Mom, "Politician?"

"Yes."

Jim, "Former president?"

"Yes, you're getting close!"

Dad, "Abraham Lincoln [his favorite president]?"

"Yes! You got it! It was too easy!"

Next, Jim challenged us with another unknown—animal, vegetable, or mineral—and the 20 questions game began anew. Each of us took turns trying to stump the others, but we rarely succeeded unless there was a breach of rules. Actually, the rules were flexible and frequently debated. In any case, after a couple of rounds, we would tire of 20 questions. Jim returned to his book, while the rest of us watched the traffic and gazed out the car windows.

Coming as we did from a sheltered middle-class suburb of Chicago, the novelties along Route 66 offered up a steady stream of distractions. Dad stopped at every historical landmark. He would slow the car to a stop, order us out, and read the commemorative plaque. In Illinois, especially, Dad was thrilled to encounter physical artifacts that connected him with his hero, Abraham Lincoln. The high point was a visit to what was said to be Lincoln's childhood home; I had seen pictures of it in a book that Dad gave me. Vladimir Nabokov, the Russian novelist, visited the same site in the period 1941–1953 when he crisscrossed America looking for rare butterflies. Later, he described the cabin in his novel, *Lolita* (1955), "The present log cabin boldly simulating the past log cabin where Lincoln was born . . . largely spurious, with parlor books and period furniture that most visitors reverently accepted as personal belongings." Dad was also adamant that we detour to Hannibal, Missouri, the home of Mark Twain between the ages of 4 and 18. He wanted to see the fence that Tom Sawyer and his friends had whitewashed. It was a rather ordinary looking fence, and I was not impressed. More intriguing, to my mind, were the vast, open stretches of cultivated fields. "What's that growing over *there*?" I asked. "It's potato," Mom would reply, or, "I'm not sure, but I *think* it's beet." Usually, though, it was corn, and even I was able to recognize corn.

Billboards were another attraction. We all jumped to attention whenever one of us spotted an approaching Burma-Shave serial advertisement:

Car in ditch / Driver in tree / Moon was full / And so / Was he /
Burma-Shave

and

I use it too / The bald man said / It keeps my face / Just like / My head
/ Burma-Shave

The restaurants where we stopped were much the same as those
where Vladimir Nabokov had eaten as he traveled on Route 66 just a few
years earlier. Humbert Humbert, the protagonist in *Lolita*, described
them well:

> [The] whole gamut of American roadside restaurants, from the lowly *Eat*
> with its deer head (dark trace of long tear at inner canthus), "humorous"
> picture post cards of the posterior "Kurort" type, impaled guest checks, life
> savers, sunglasses, adman visions of celestial sundaes, one half of a choc-
> olate cake under glass, and several horribly experienced flies zigzagging
> over the sticky sugar-pour on the ignoble counter; all the way to the expen-
> sive place with the subdued lights, preposterously poor table linen, inept
> waiters . . .

Choosing lodging for the night was more contentious. Jim and I preferred motels displaying decayed wagon wheels or other relics of the
imagined past, whereas Mom put the emphasis on quiet, comfort, and
cleanliness. Dad was not fussy except that he, like the rest of us, liked to
dip into a swimming pool after a long day on the road. We took our clues
of quality from the signage. If the signs were neatly painted and showed
some originality, Dad would pull over for a closer look. Sometimes we
would have a heated debate about the merits of a particular establishment, but in the end, each new motel closely resembled the previous
one. Occasionally, Dad treated us to something out of the ordinary. I
recall one place that could well have been the Chestnut Court, also visited by Lolita and Humbert Humbert, "nice cabins, damp green grounds,
apple trees, an old swing—and a tremendous sunset which the tired
child [Lolita] ignored."

We dipped south into exotic Oklahoma, Texas, and New Mexico.
While Dad reveled in the historical sites marking battlegrounds and

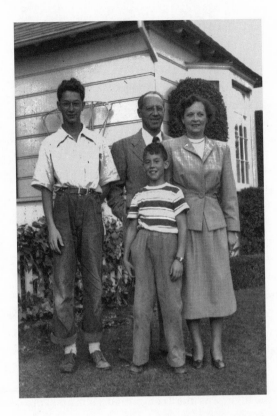

**Jim with his family
outside their new home
in Los Angeles, 1948**

exploration routes, I was fascinated by the dry wastelands. The heat
scorched our throats, and the wind blew dust into the car. We dropped
coins into the soft drink machines at gas stations, where a selection of
colorful bottles stood upright in icy baths, among which were the exciting Dr. Pepper and the refreshing lime-flavored sodas. Driving through
a small town in Texas, Dad's vision became obscured by a cloud of
swarming locusts. He pulled to the side of the road, and Mom stepped
gingerly out of the car. She slipped on insect bodies, shrieked, and dove
back inside. We stopped at so many reptile zoos that Dad finally said
enough, we cannot stop at any more. However, to encourage my interest
in nature, he allowed me to capture a horned toad. I cared for that toad
all the way to Los Angeles, where it died.

Neither Mom nor Dad had told us what to expect in the deserts
of New Mexico and Arizona, probably because they didn't know

themselves. But for me, this was the best part of the trip. The intense heat enveloped the forsaken homesteads and the rusted machinery; huge bundles of tumbleweed blew across the highway, darting between soft drink signs. Farther along, after passing through the towns of Daggett, Barstow, and Oro Grande, we encountered our first citrus groves in San Bernardino. Finally, Southern California. Two weeks on the road had brought us to our destination, and everyone felt the excitement of a new life opening before us.

Exactly 50 years later, as Jim was nearing the end of his life, he and I were engaged in an unusually frank conversation. We were reminiscing about the old times before he became ill. When I mentioned the road trip on Route 66, he paused to refresh his memories. Then, speaking with a serious voice, he asked, "How did Dad do it? How did he find the way?"

2

Who Gets Schizophrenia and Why?

None of us had even an inkling, no reason whatsoever to anticipate that Jim would develop schizophrenia, but once it became clear that he was suffering from the illness, the questions inevitably arose. What happened? Why did Jim, of all people, get schizophrenia? Desperate though we were to answer these questions, we found no help in the philosophical or religious beliefs that bring comfort to some families. It was not enough to say that Jim's illness was due to fate or God's will. We—my parents and I—needed an explanation based on facts in this world. And so, a few years after Jim became a person with schizophrenia, I became a scientist. I began gathering information about schizophrenia. Here is what I learned.

Schizophrenia is often described with reference to two categories of symptoms. The so-called positive symptoms are not ordinarily found in healthy individuals; the most prominent are hallucinations (usually auditory), delusions (often paranoid), disorganized speech, and **disorganized behavior**. The so-called negative symptoms involve normal attributes that are weakened or absent in people with schizophrenia; they include poverty of thought, reduced **affect**, reduced ambition, and few social interactions. Untreated individuals with schizophrenia have both positive and negative symptoms, although the specific symptoms vary from person to person. Therapies are much more likely to moderate the positive symptoms than to alleviate the negative symptoms.

It is often stated that schizophrenia affects 1 in 100 individuals, but a recent study estimates that the **prevalence** is closer to 7 individuals per 1,000, or 0.7 per 100.[1] The figure is a measure of the lifetime prevalence of schizophrenia, or the chance that a person will get the disease during the entire course of his or her life.[2] Schizophrenia is a disease that affects people around the world regardless of race, social class, or economic circumstance. That said, city dwellers are more likely to have the disease than people living in rural areas, and people living at high latitudes are more likely to have schizophrenia than people living near the equator. Other data indicate that schizophrenia is especially prevalent among individuals who have moved from one country to another and that there might also be ethnic differences.

Although there are good reasons to accept these statistical data as reflecting something real, their interpretation is anything but straightforward. Epidemiologists suspect that it is not city living, migration, or high latitude, as such, that accounts for the high rates of schizophrenia, but something else that happens to be associated with those factors. For example, city dwellers and migrants may be more prone to infectious diseases, economic hardship, or other types of stress. According to another hypothesis, people living at high latitudes may be vulnerable because they do not get enough vitamin D (because of limited exposures to sunlight). Later in the book, I will discuss these and other hypotheses.

For biologists, schizophrenia is a trait, which simply means that it is a characteristic, or feature, present in at least some members of the species. Although arguments rage over which traits are due to "nature," meaning heredity, and which are due to "nurture," meaning the **environment**, the truth is that virtually all traits in all animals (including humans) are shaped by *both* heredity (**genes**) and the environment. Schizophrenia is no exception to this rule. And yet, how do we know that both genes and the environment play a role in schizophrenia, and what proportion of cause can be assigned to each?

I once had the pleasure of conducting research at the Max Planck Institute for Psychiatry in Munich, Germany. In the nineteenth century, the psychiatrist Emil Kraepelin worked at the hospital that is located at the same site. (In recognition of his important contributions to the understanding of schizophrenia and other mental illnesses, the street has been named Kraepelinstrasse.) Ernst Rüdin, one of Kraepelin's department heads at the Munich hospital, conducted a study to determine whether schizophrenia is inherited. His main finding, published in 1916, and later replicated by many other investigators, was that schizophrenia runs in families. Today, nearly everyone knows this. My parents and I knew it. Yet none of us had schizophrenia and, to the best of our knowledge, there had been no schizophrenia in either my mother's family or my father's family. Indeed, in the majority of schizophrenia cases, there is no family history of the disease. More than 90 percent of people with schizophrenia have neither a mother nor a father who has schizophrenia, and about 60 percent of people who have schizophrenia have no first- or second-degree relative with the disorder. Nevertheless, Rüdin got it right in his original study: overall, there is more clustering of schizophrenia in families than one would expect by chance.

Just because schizophrenia runs in families does not necessarily mean that it is transmitted by genes. Other explanations might include cultural practices, infections, and learned behaviors. Scientists sort out these possibilities by taking a close look at the patterns of family transmission. From basic genetic principles, we know that a person's first-degree relatives (parents, children, and siblings) share more genes in common with that individual than do second-degree relatives (aunts, uncles, nieces, and nephews), who, in turn, share more genes with the individual than do third-degree relatives (first cousins). Therefore, if the risk of schizophrenia is transmitted through genes, one would expect that the highest number of cases would show up in the first-degree relatives of persons with schizophrenia, followed by the second-degree relatives; the third-degree relatives would have the fewest number of cases.

To test this prediction, groups of geneticists, working independently from one another in several countries, located thousands of people who were relatives of people with schizophrenia. By and large, the results confirm the predictions—that is, schizophrenia is more prevalent in first-degree relatives than in second-degree relatives, and more prevalent in second-degree relatives than in third-degree relatives. For example, when the relatives of people with schizophrenia are tracked down, 13 percent of the children, 5 percent of the grandchildren, and only 2 percent of the first cousins are found to have schizophrenia.

While these results support the idea that schizophrenia is hereditary, they are not sufficient to prove it. Additional support comes from adoption studies and twin studies.[3]

Adoption studies provide a means of testing whether the family influence is due to genes or the home environment. Early studies looked at what happens to children who are at risk of schizophrenia because a parent has the disease. Children who were raised by their biological parents (one of whom had schizophrenia) were compared with children who were raised by adoptive parents (none of whom had a psychiatric illness). If the family influence is primarily due to genes, one would expect that being raised in an adoptive family would not reduce the risk of schizophrenia, and this is what most studies find. However, for practical reasons, it is difficult to find enough cases to draw firm conclusions from this type of study.

An alternative approach looks only at adopted children who develop schizophrenia, and it asks whether, on the whole, there is more schizophrenia in the biological families or in the adoptive families. The big advantage of this approach is that the test cases can be easily found in national registries. For example, when investigators in Denmark searched a national registry of 14,500 adoptions from the years 1924 to 1947, they found that 74 of the adopted children had developed schizophrenia. A telling result was obtained when the investigators then examined the medical records of the parents of these children who developed schizophrenia. They learned that 21.4 percent of the biological parents had schizophrenia or a related illness, whereas only 5.4 percent of the adoptive parents had these same illnesses. Therefore, because schizophrenia was more strongly associated with the biological parents than with the adoptive parents, and because the children had been placed in their adoptive homes at a very young age, it is reasonable to conclude that the main cause of their illnesses was the genes that they had inherited from their biological parents.

Another adoption study points to an interaction between genes and the environment. Here, two groups of Finnish adoptees were studied.[4] The children in one group were considered to be at high risk for getting schizophrenia because their biological mothers had schizophrenia, whereas the children in the second, control, group were considered to be at low risk because their biological mothers had no major psychiatric disorder. Psychiatric investigators then went into the adopted homes not knowing the risk status of the children. They observed each family for two full days, and they interviewed family members. From the information gathered, they scored the quality of family functioning by measuring such factors as communication, conflict, and levels of emotional expression. Much later, the investigators determined which kids had developed schizophrenia.

The most interesting results in this study pertain to the high-genetic-risk adoptees, where it was found that the risk of getting schizophrenia depended on the environment in the adopted home. If the child was raised in a "healthy" family, the lifetime risk was 5.8 percent, whereas it was 36.8 percent if the child was raised in a "dysfunctional" family. We can conclude from this study that the genetic risk carried by a child from his or her parent who has schizophrenia is reduced—but not eliminated—when the child is raised in a healthy environment. Genes are important, but they are not everything. I will have more to say about gene-environment interactions later, but now turn to studies of twins. Twin studies allow scientists to measure the relative sizes of the genetic and environmental contributions.

As everyone knows, twins are of two types. In most cases, each twin comes from a separate fertilized egg; these twins are called dizygotic, meaning from two eggs. More rarely, a single fertilized egg divides to yield two eggs and two offspring; these are monozygotic twins. There is a crucial biological distinction between the types because the twins in a monozygotic pair have exactly the same genes—hence the name *identical twins*—whereas in dizygotic pairs only half of the genes are identical—hence, *fraternal twins*.[5] The identical pairs are interesting for psychiatric geneticists because they allow for a simple test of a key hypothesis. If genes are completely responsible for who gets schizophrenia, then finding schizophrenia in one member of an identical pair should lead investigators to find schizophrenia in the other twin.

Some psychiatric researchers did the experiment. They started by locating an identical twin who had schizophrenia. Next, they located the other member of the pair in order to calculate the **concordance**, which is the percentage of cases (rate) in which *both* of the twins have schizophrenia. Some studies conducted in the period 1928–1961 found concordance rates of about 60 percent, on average. The problem is, the sample sizes were very small in these studies, for obvious reasons, so the results were not necessarily reliable. What the researchers needed was a much larger database. They seized on the strategy of looking into the medical registries of entire nations. In Denmark, they obtained a list of 7,000 same-sex pairs; in the United States, they used a registry containing 15,924 twin pairs (both identical and fraternal), all of whom were male veterans of the armed forces. Using sophisticated investigative and statistical methods, these modern studies found concordance rates of about 50 percent for identical twins, thus generally confirming the earlier results.[6] In five smaller, more recent studies, the concordance rate for identical twins ranged from 41 percent to 65 percent or, again, roughly 50 percent. Contrasting with this, the rate for fraternal twins ranged from 0 to 28 percent in recent studies.[7]

The 50 percent concordance rate for identical twins is striking, and it immediately suggests a genetic basis for schizophrenia.[8] The difference between the high concordances for identical twins and the relatively low concordances for fraternal twins is also very interesting. Twins, regardless of type, are usually raised together, so they share much of the same environment. Nevertheless, the concordance rates are different for the identical twins and the fraternal twins. Because the environments are very similar in both cases, the different concordance rates must be attributed to the fact that identical twins share all their genes, whereas fraternal twins share only half of their genes. Yet genetics cannot be solely responsible for schizophrenia, because the concordance for identical twins would be 100 percent if that were true.

Twin studies can also be used to determine the portions of responsibility for schizophrenia that can be assigned to genetics and to the environment. Researchers compare the rates of concordance for the two types of twins, identical and fraternal, and their analysis yields a numerical factor, called **heritability**, which represents the proportion of the risk for schizophrenia, that can be assigned to genetic factors.[9] The calculated heritability for schizophrenia turns out to be approximately 80 percent, which means that the remaining 20 percent of risk is due to the environment. While it satisfying to be able to put numbers on the sources of risk, it is important to understand exactly what heritability means.

First, because the estimate is based on combined data from many different twins, its assignments of responsibility apply only to populations, not to any individual persons; the influences of genetics and the environment varies from one person to another. Second, and this point follows from the preceding one, the figure of 80 percent heritability says that 80 percent of the *variability in risk* is due to *variability in heredity*; it does not imply that genetics is 80 percent of the cause. This is a subtle, but important, distinction. Finally, one should bear in mind that the concordance rates for twin pairs are facts derived from surveys, whereas the heritability value is a theoretical estimate derived from the factual data. In other words, the concordance rates are indisputable, whereas the heritability values are only as good as the underlying assumptions.

Heritability can be estimated for any human trait. If we compare schizophrenia with other psychiatric diseases, we find that bipolar disease is equally heritable, at about 80 percent, whereas autism appears to be more highly heritable, at around 90 percent, and major depression is less heritable at 40 percent. The human trait that has been most intensively studied is body height. The heritability of human height differences is similar to that for schizophrenia, approximately 80 percent, implying that most of the variation in height is due to variation in genes. Significant differences in height heritability exist between countries and across time. Most likely, the inconsistent values reflect the fact that a person's ultimate height is dependent, in part, on his or her history of nutrition and disease, both of which are strongly influenced by economic conditions. The heritability of intelligence (IQ) steadily increases with age as the child's environment becomes increasingly matched to his or her genetic endowment, thereby reducing the variability of the environmental component. For adults, the heritability of intelligence ranges from 50 to 80 percent according to different estimates. Altogether, heritability has been estimated for several thousand human traits. Here are some more: birth weight, 10 percent; smoking, 35 percent for females, 70 percent for males; participation in sports, 50 percent.

Ultimately, we would like to identify the specific genes and the specific environmental factors that create the risk of schizophrenia, for only then will it be possible to design truly effective measures to combat the disease. In subsequent chapters, I will review progress toward these goals.

SUMMARY

- Schizophrenia affects about 7 persons in 1,000. Although everyone is potentially at risk, members of certain groups seem especially vulnerable, including migrants, urban dwellers, and people living at high latitudes.

- Genetics plays a significant role in who gets schizophrenia. Family studies demonstrate that the close relatives of people with schizophrenia are more likely to get the disease than are distant relatives. The hereditary basis of the disease is further indicated by studies of adopted children, although these same studies also show that a good environment can attenuate the inherited risk.

- Twin studies provide the strongest evidence for a genetic contribution. Schizophrenia is much more likely to appear in both members of a pair of identical twins, who share 100 percent of their genes, than in both members of a fraternal pair, who share only about 50 percent of their genes. Even so, in about half of the identical pairs with schizophrenia, one twin has the disease but the other does not, thus proving that genetics is not the sole cause.

- Medical geneticists use the data from twin studies to calculate the heritability of schizophrenia. They estimate that 80 percent of the variation for the risk of schizophrenia comes from variation in genes; the remaining 20 percent comes from variations in the environment. Thus, both genes (nature) and the environment (nurture) contribute to schizophrenia, which happens to be true for every other trait in every species of animals.

- Neither "bad" genes alone nor "bad" environments alone are sufficient to cause schizophrenia. Exactly how the environment and the genes interact remains an open question, but it is unlikely to be a matter of simple addition.

3

Dining with Tension

In Los Angeles, we settled into a comfortable home on a quiet street near the UCLA campus. A few years later, Jim was completing his undergraduate studies in English literature at UCLA. I was attending a nearby high school. Jim was a serious student, and I was preoccupied with competitive running more than with my coursework. One evening, I had come home late from school following an exceptionally long training session on the running track. I was relaxing in my room, and Jim was in his room, probably reading. Dad was busy going over some papers he had brought home from work. Each of us heard the *ting-a-ling-a-ling* of the small stainless steel bell that Mom used to call the family to dinner. "Dinner time!" she shouted out. She took little pleasure in cooking, but as a full-time mother and a homemaker she had little option but to prepare the family meals. She generally rotated through a few standards: roast beef with potatoes, brisket (lots of ketchup), chicken soup, macaroni and cheese, and occasionally fish. Sometimes she would mix things up with a Jewish dish such as matzo ball soup, kasha, or blintzes. On this evening, it was meatloaf covered with strips of fatty bacon.

At the center of our cozy dining room stood an ordinary wooden table surrounded by four straight-backed chairs. An ornate chandelier hung above. Mom sat near the kitchen at one end, Dad sat at the other end, and Jim and I sat opposite each other in the middle. Looming behind Jim was a lovely pine hutch holding Mom's precious dinnerware.

As soon as I sat down, I knew that we were bound for trouble. There had been a time when we could look forward to dinner as an occasion

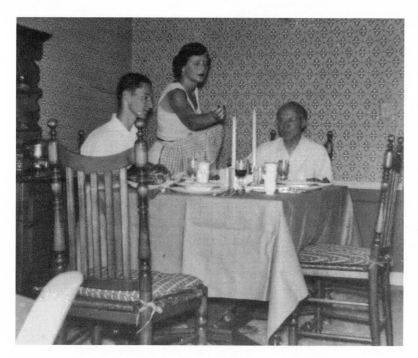

Jim, his mother, and his father at dinner, 1955

for discussing everything from world events to family affairs. It was a time to relax after a hard day at school or at the office. Of late, however, our dinners had become more stressful than relaxing. I looked at Jim and saw that his head was bent downward so far that it nearly touched his chest. His tight facial muscles were a sure sign that he would not be engaging in light chatter.

Sizing up the situation, I decided that it would be safest to ignore Jim. I turned to Mom and said, "Sorry, Mom, but I can't eat the potatoes tonight. I told you, I'm running the half mile in our track meet on Friday, and I want to beat Al Gentry. Coach says you're supposed to lay off carbohydrates for a day or two before a race, and then stuff yourself with pasta in your last meal before the race. I'm not going to have any carbohydrates either tonight or tomorrow. At lunch on Friday, I'll pig-out on spaghetti in the cafeteria. I'm also taking extra large doses of wheat germ oil."

"Sit up, Jim!" Dad blurted out. We all stiffened in our chairs as Dad spoke, but Jim did not move as ordered.

"Didn't you hear me? *Sit up!*"

Mom joined in, "Jimmie, dear, please do as your father asks."

Slowly, Jim straightened up, but he continued to look down at his plate. The rest of us attempted to carry on a normal conversation. "Ronnie, I know you are going to do well on Friday," said Mom. "Once you put your mind to it, you can do anything."

"What do you know?" I shouted out in a voice made loud by the tension. "I didn't do so great last week when I ran the quarter mile at Hollywood High, did I? You're only saying that to make me feel good, not because it's really true."

"Oh, please Ronnie, there's no reason to raise your voice. I am only trying to encourage you. If you believe that you will run fast, you will. And besides, you said that you've been training hard."

Mom then turned to Jim, who had hardly touched his food. Naturally tall and thin, Jim had become even thinner in recent weeks.

"What's bothering you, dear? Please, *please* eat something. Don't you like the meatloaf?"

Jim didn't answer. Instead, he again lowered his head and began to rock his body back and forth in a slow, deliberate rhythm. Mom softly pleaded while Dad and I sat transfixed. We were all anxious because we recognized, from previous experiences, the signs of a pending disaster. First there would be a fuss about getting Jim to come to the table; he sometimes refused to come out from behind his barred door despite our pleadings. And when he did join us at the table, we had to wait to see whether he would say anything; he could sit through an entire meal without saying a single word. Inevitably, on these tense occasions, some remark by one of us would set Jim off on a violent outburst.

On this evening, Jim sat stone-faced and motionless except for the rocking. Mom attempted to placate and soothe him, but Dad interrupted by asking Jim to pass the salt. Jim paid no notice to Dad's request.

"Jim, I asked you, would you *please* pass the salt!" Still nothing.

"What is the matter with you!" shouted Dad as he banged his fist on the table. And then it started for real.

"*Why can't you just leave me alone!*" shouted Jim in his loudest, most angry voice.

Mom pitched in, "Jim, dear, what *is* the matter? We want to help you . . ."

"Just leave me alone," Jim repeated, this time more softly, in a plaintive voice.

"Now dear . . ."

I said nothing while this was going on because I was afraid of triggering the final explosion. We all knew where this was headed, but none of us knew how to forestall it. Dad was particularly befuddled. All he could think of was the salt.

"Jim, I'm still waiting for the salt." Too late, as it turned out.

Instantly, Jim bolted from his chair and launched his fork across the table. The fork hit my glass of milk, which spilled onto my lap. Then Jim took a swipe at his own glass, sending a white blur in Dad's direction. Wordless screams came out of Jim's mouth as he hurried around the table, crossed the hallway, and ran into his room. The sound of his door slamming shut marked the tremulous termination of our family dinner. We other three picked up the broken glass and dabbed at the wet spots on our clothing. And then, as if it were someone's fault, the accusations and the recriminations began.

Mom: "*You see what you did, Joe!* Every time you speak to him like that, he flies off in a rage. If you knew better how to behave toward your son, maybe these things would not happen."

Dad: "What? Me? You're blaming *me* for this when it is *you* who coddles him? So far as you're concerned, he can do whatever he wants. You don't seem to care whether he sits up straight or slumps, whether he responds to polite requests or ignores us. At some point, we've got to say to him, 'Enough already. It's time for you to grow up and act like an adult.'"

Mom: "Well, he's your son too. You can at least treat him as though you love him, even if you don't."

Dad: "What do you mean, I don't love him? I love him just as much as you do. I am only trying to get him to behave like an adult. I don't understand what's wrong with him. We've given him everything: a nice bedroom, money for all the books he wants, even money for a car that he does not want. My goodness, most boys his age have after-school jobs, but not our son. You'd think that he could at least behave like a normal human being around here. It's getting so bad that I don't look forward to our dinners any more. And, none of this can be good for Ronnie either."

Mom: "I'll tell you what's wrong with Jim. *It's you.* How do you expect him to behave properly, to do what you tell him to do, when he doesn't respect you? Let's face it, Joe, you're a weakling. Instead of setting a strong example, you send him confusing messages. One day you tolerate his poor manners and lack of communication, dismissing it as part of his so-called intellectual personality, and then the next day, you lash out at him for the same behavior."

Dad: "No, No. Again, you've got it backward. It's not me who is inconsistent, it's *you.*"

And so it went. Having heard similar arguments before, and sensitized to their crushing effect on my own moods, I went to work clearing dishes from the table. Once I had finished that task, I retired to my room to do homework. With Jim in his bedroom and me in mine, Mom and Dad were free to continue their bitter exchanges without fear of interference, but their harsh voices, if not their exact words, resounded through the house. It took me about an hour to complete my homework. I was still feeling badly about what had happened at dinner so I knocked gently on Jim's door. Jim was often receptive to me at times when he was angry with Mom and Dad. I was not surprised, therefore, when he opened the door and let me in. His was a small room with a bed, a desk, a reading chair, and a bookcase. He kept it tidy. The bed, for example, was always made up and covered with a bedspread. For some reason, I felt that the chairs were more exclusively his than was the bed, so I sat down on the bed.

"What are you reading?" I asked.

"*Gulliver's Travels* by Jonathan Swift. I don't suppose you've read it yet, but you should. Swift is maybe the greatest novelist of all time, and this is his most famous book. It's about a fellow, Gulliver, who travels to imaginary countries where he encounters all sorts of strange things. But the entire story is satirical. Swift's purpose was to criticize British politics and British morals. The book itself is incredibly funny and modern despite the fact that it was published in 1726. It's a masterpiece of English literature." Before I could respond, he started reading a passage from the book,

> They go on shore to rob and plunder, they see a harmless people, are entertained with kindness; they give the country a new name; they take formal possession of it for their king; they set up a rotten plank, or a stone, for a memorial; they murder two or three dozen of the natives, bring away a couple more, by force, for a sample; return home, and get their pardon. Here commences a new dominion acquired with a title by divine right. Ships are sent with the first opportunity; the natives driven out or destroyed; their princes tortured to discover their gold; a free license given to all acts of inhumanity and lust, the earth reeking with the blood of its inhabitants . . .

"What do you suppose Swift is writing about in this passage?" Jim asked.

"Well," I stumbled, "I don't really know. The language is odd; I suppose the author is describing Gulliver's visit to an exotic island."

"You forget, the story takes place more than 200 years ago. Swift is writing about colonialism, at a time when England was establishing its empire in North America, the Caribbean, and Asia. You see, his description of the colonialists' activities is satirical, even humorous, but he jolts us with his reference to 'the earth reeking with the blood of the inhabitants.' Swift is brilliant, just brilliant."

I had never before heard of Jonathan Swift, let alone read any of his books, whereas Jim was studying Swift in one of his classes at UCLA. He spent a lot of time reading. He read huge, thick books on school assignments, but he also read many other works that he himself chose. He consumed classical English poetry (Chaucer, Milton, Pope), early novels (Cervantes, Austin, Hardy), and contemporary literature (Roth, Huxley, Isherwood). Literature was his refuge, one might say, a place where he could go to quiet his mind. The printed words were defined and interpretable, whereas the turbulent thoughts in his mind were not.

After listening to a few more morsels from Swift, I grew tired of him. "Would you like to play a game of chess?" I asked.

"Sure," Jim replied, "but it's getting late. Unless I mate you quickly, we'll have to finish tomorrow."

"Okay, let's go. I'll set up the board."

Jim and I enjoyed a healthy competition in games. We mostly played board games because Jim wasn't much of an athlete, but we occasionally played ping pong, and we shot basketballs at the net that Dad installed above the garage door. We played Monopoly for fun, but checkers, and especially chess, were serious affairs. Although Jim was definitely the better chess player (he even had a book of strategies), I became good enough to scare him on occasion. That night, however, Jim led me into a couple of traps and beat me easily. Clearly, he was feeling better now that his psychic demons had retreated, even if only temporarily. We wished each other a good night, and I returned to my room.

Dinners like this one had occurred before that evening, and they repeated themselves in the following weeks and months. Jim's outbursts came more often and became more violent. There were other signs that all was not well with my brother. He spent an increasing amount of time in his room behind the closed door, and he absented himself from more meals. His conversations, once articulate and peppered with witticisms, became short and shallow. We were all suffering, but no one knew how to relieve the tensions. Jim, for his part, did not tell us what was troubling him. Maybe he was embarrassed to say, or maybe he did not know himself. Later, I learned that a hallmark of psychosis is the inability to recognize the difference between subjective consciousness and the objective, external world. I think Jim did not talk to us because the boundary between the two realities was beginning to crumble.

4

Which Genes Cause Schizophrenia?

It would be nearly 20 years before I realized that the family tensions of my adolescent years were anything but ordinary. In my naiveté, I assumed that people in every home were shouting at each other, throwing things, and pounding tables. I thought it was normal for kids to insult their parents, imprison themselves in their rooms, and refuse to engage in simple conversations. My family knew nothing about mental illness because no one in either my mother's family or my father's family had any serious mental problems. Yes, from the printed media and from television we vaguely knew of "crazy people" living in "insane asylums," but those were stories of *other people*; certainly, nothing of the sort would happen to *us*. We were healthy, educated, and middle class. We were busy advancing our personal agendas, whether social, economic, or athletic. Likewise, we knew little about science, and again, it would be many years before I realized this. Each of us knew that the Irish author James Joyce had written a celebrated novel called *Ulysses*, but none of us knew that the structure of deoxyribonucleic acid had been discovered as recently as 1953. I do not think that we even knew about genes.

Gregor Mendel, a nineteenth-century monk from Silesia in the Austrian Empire, was the first person to demonstrate that traits are transmitted from one generation to the next through physical entities, later identified as genes. From his research on pea plants, and that of others who followed him, we have come to suspect genes in the causation of any disease found to be inherited from one's parents or clustered in extended families. The chemical nature of genes was discovered by James

Watson and Francis Crick in 1953.[1] Mendel was fortunate in that the traits that he studied, primarily the colors of pea plant flowers, are wholly determined by a single gene. Several thousand human traits are also transmitted by single genes, including albinism, cleft chin, and face freckles; these are known as Mendelian traits. As well, a few dozen human diseases are of the Mendelian variety, including Huntington's disease, cystic fibrosis, and retinoblastoma.

Mendelian diseases can be recognized by their characteristic patterns of inheritance in families. Two patterns are giveaways. With the *dominance* pattern, when either of the parents has the disease, 50 percent of the children get it. Because the risk of schizophrenia is only 13 percent when one parent has the disease, it is clearly not inherited through a dominant gene. Things become more complicated if one imagines that a disease is inherited through a *recessive* gene and only one parent has the disease,[2] but if *both* parents have the disease, then 100 percent of the children will get it. Studies show, however, that when both parents have schizophrenia, fewer than half of the offspring get schizophrenia. So, one can say with certainty that, even though schizophrenia is partly inherited, it is not caused by a **mutation** in any single gene.[3] Instead, schizophrenia is one of many inherited medical conditions that are caused by multiple gene mutations; doctors call these diseases "complex."

In addition to schizophrenia, the complex diseases include most of the cancers, Parkinson's disease, Alzheimer's disease, and multiple sclerosis. All of these illnesses occur at rates exceeding two cases per 1,000 persons, making them much more common than any Mendelian disease. Each of the complex diseases is believed to be caused by a large number of genes. In the case of schizophrenia, one recent investigation concludes that *thousands* of genes determine the risk of getting the disease, with each individual gene contributing just a small effect.[4] Because the risk is expected to increase with the number of mutant genes carried by an individual, the more family members who have schizophrenia, the greater should be the risk for that individual, and the evidence seems to bear this out.

Genes are nothing but segments of **DNA**. Every gene produces a **protein**, and the chemical composition of that protein depends on the specific sequence of DNA "letters" within the segment. The human **genome** is estimated to contain about 23,000 genes together with large sequences of DNA that do not code for protein but have either regulatory roles or unknown functions. The entire sequence of letters in the genome of a single individual was determined for the first time in 2001, a milestone achievement that took several years of intense work and many millions of dollars. By contrast, investigators today can sequence a person's genome in one day for about $3,000, and the cost continues to go down.

Although there is more than one way to search for the genes that confer the risk for schizophrenia, the most common method simply compares the genomes of people with schizophrenia with those of people who have no psychiatric illness. Ordinarily, it is not necessary to read every single letter in the DNA code, because there are shortcuts. If a mutation appears in a higher proportion of the disease-affected cases than in the disease-free cases, the mutated gene is said to be associated with the disease, and it becomes a candidate risk factor for the disease. Investigations of this type are known as genome-wide association studies.

It is not possible to specify exactly how many genes have been identified in these studies. One review of the literature, published in 2012, focused on genes that have a highly significant statistical association with schizophrenia, were documented in research involving a minimum of 20,000 subjects (patients plus normal controls), and were replicated in multiple studies.[5] Seventeen genes satisfied these criteria. However, new associations are still being discovered. And, by simply relaxing the statistical criteria, many more genes could be added to the list. Indeed, the authors of the review article believe that "hundreds" of different genes contribute to the risk of schizophrenia. Medical experts and psychiatric researchers refer to the strongly associated genes as the "risk genes" for schizophrenia.[6]

Here is a short sample of known risk genes: *NRGN* makes neurogranin, a protein that is found in **synapses**; *COMT* makes an enzyme that degrades (inactivates) several key **neurotransmitters**; *ZNF804A* makes a protein that activates other genes; and *CACNA1C* makes a voltage-sensitive channel in nerve cell membranes. In addition to the risk genes that operate mainly or exclusively in the brain, many genes with roles in immunity are implicated; these genes form part of the major histocompatibility complex (MHC). Others genes make proteins with roles in metabolism and gene regulation. The functions of still other candidate risk genes have yet to be determined.

Knowing the genes that are involved in schizophrenia can open the door to major advances in our scientific understanding of the disease. Because every gene has a specific function, once a gene has been implicated in schizophrenia, the spotlight of further research can focus on the biological process that is likely affected by the mutation. A large proportion of the risk genes that have so far been identified in genome-wide association studies make proteins that control the development of the brain, from its earliest embryonic stages through to late adolescence. This finding has encouraged neuroscience researchers to think about the structural and physiological abnormalities that can result from improper brain development, as I describe in chapter 12.

This kind of knowledge can lead to effective treatments for people who have schizophrenia. In addition, knowing the genetic signature that puts people at risk for schizophrenia can help doctors identify those individuals who are likely to develop the disease. If the identification is done at an early age, measures might be taken to either block or reverse the developmental defects that lead to a full expression of the disease. I hasten to point out, however, that we are far from achieving these goals today. Despite the impressive achievements of recent years, we still do not know enough about the genetics of schizophrenia to create practical applications. Blocking the way toward more rapid progress is the complex nature of schizophrenia genetics and the brute reality of statistics, as I will explain.

Researchers disagree about exactly which genes, or even which types of genes, cause schizophrenia. According to one view, the culpable genes (actually, **gene variants**, or mutated genes) are relatively common in the total human population, and they ordinarily produce no ill effects. It is only when they appear in combination with many other risk genes that trouble arises. In this scenario, no gene, by itself, is sufficient to cause schizophrenia, nor is any particular gene required to be part of the mix that causes schizophrenia. Therefore, no researcher should expect to find a gene that is mutated in every person with schizophrenia but in no person who does not have schizophrenia.

The findings to date confirm this view because even the most highly ranked risk genes are associated with increases in schizophrenia amounting to just one case for every 1,000 persons carrying the mutation. Thus, knowing ahead of time that an individual has a risk gene does not significantly increase the accuracy of predicting whether that person will get schizophrenia. Even the combined predictive power of *all* the currently known risk genes accounts for only a small fraction of the total heritability of schizophrenia. This means that even if a person has all the currently identified risk genes, the chances of getting schizophrenia are slim.

It is also disconcerting to learn that different genome-wide association studies identify different risk genes. This might be due, in part, to the use of different investigative methods. However, it could also be the case that schizophrenia requires only a minimum number of gene variants, and if one risk variant is absent in a particular individual, another variant from a different risk gene can "substitute" for it. If so, different combinations of gene variants would create risk in different individuals. Further complicating things is that some genes have powerful effects on the activities of other genes,[7] so depending on which genes are in the mix, a few gene variants that interact strongly with each other may be more decisive than a large number of mutated, but noninteracting, genes. Finally, another probable cause of discrepant results lies in the uncertain definition of schizophrenia itself. Whereas we tend to think of it as a single disease, it is more likely a family of related diseases, each with its own clinical characteristics and its own genetic constitution.[8] Therefore, the genetics of one research sample may look very different from that of another sample, depending on how many cases of a certain type of schizophrenia are represented in each sample.

Apart from the problem of inconsistent results, a statistical barrier stands in the way of more productive genome-wide association studies. To understand this problem, imagine that you want to find genes affecting the heights of humans. You conduct a genome-wide association study using 10 tall people and 10 short people, and you find that 8 of the

10 tall individuals have a certain variant X, whereas only 6 of the 10 short individuals have variant X. Should you conclude that variant X is influential in making people tall? I think not, because the result could be just a statistical fluke. But, if you were to conduct another genome-wide association study, this time scanning the genomes of 100,000 people in each height class and finding that 81,136 tall people had the variant whereas only 62,081 short people had it, *then* you would be justified in concluding that the gene is involved. The size of the sample matters a lot when interpreting the results of any survey, whether it is estimating the distribution of human genes or the prevalence of human opinions.

The role of the variant can also be critical in determining the required sample size: the smaller the influence of a gene variant, or the rarer the variant, the larger the sample size must be to detect its effect. A useful example is human height variation, as becomes evident using numbers from a real investigation.[9] Human height, like the risk of schizophrenia, is about 80 percent heritable. In one recent study, 180 genes were found to be involved in determining human height.[10] Because each gene alone has only a small effect on height, though, the genomes of nearly 185,000 individuals had to be analyzed to obtain statistical significance for all 180 genes. Even more discouraging is that, after combining the influence of all 180 genes, this total accounts for just 10 percent of the variation in height that can be explained by heredity. The authors of the study found evidence suggesting the involvement of another 517 genes, which would boost to 16 percent the amount of variability in height that could be explained by heredity, but to find these additional genes would require examining the genomes of *another 500,000 persons*. Here we come to the crux of the problem. To obtain half a million schizophrenia cases for a study of genetic risk using methods similar to those used in the height study would be extremely expensive and time-consuming, given the relatively low prevalence of the disease (seven cases in 1,000 persons), the small number of affected people available for study, and the necessity for informed consent. In short, collecting enough schizophrenia cases to reach the level of statistical significance necessary to discover genes of small effect may not be possible.

In light of the failure, so far, to identify all the genes responsible for the inheritance of schizophrenia, height, and many other complex traits, some authors speak of a "case of missing heritability." Others refer to the genes responsible for complex traits as the "dark matter" of the human genome, with reference to the cosmic stuff that is presumed to exist on the evidence of stellar gravitational measurements but has not yet been seen. One commentator admits that, "even when dozens of genes have been linked to a trait, both the individual and cumulative effects are disappointingly small and nowhere near enough to explain . . . estimates of heritability."[11] To fill the theoretical gap, several new ideas for explaining the heritability of complex traits have come to light, and the field of medical genetics is churning with more discussion and more DNA analyses than ever before. All the leading hypotheses challenge the idea that the genetic risk for schizophrenia is entirely due to the accumulation of a large number of common gene variants, each of which alone has just a small effect. Let's take a brief look at the alternative hypotheses.

Many geneticists think that more attention should be paid to the possibility that certain rare mutations may have highly potent effects and that each such mutation, acting either alone or with a small number of other rare mutations, has the ability to substantially increase the risk for schizophrenia. The postulated role of rare mutations need not be seen as an exclusive alternative to that of common gene variants but rather as a complementary scenario. Rare mutations are usually missed in genome-wide association studies because, for reasons of efficiency, only the most common gene variants are detected, typically those present in at least 1 percent of the population. Newer methods, however, permit a more detailed, more in-depth examination of the human genome, and they are revealing some startling facts. It turns out that 86 percent of all gene variants (including, but not limited to, those responsible for schizophrenia) occur in less than 0.5 percent of the population; in other words, most variants are rare.[12] On average, research shows, each person carries 13,595 variants measured at the level of single DNA "letters," and, again on average, 2.3 percent of these variants are expected to affect the function of proteins in deleterious ways. Ordinarily, harmful genes are eliminated from the genome by evolution acting through the mechanism of natural selection. Why these (potentially) harmful gene variants are still hanging around is because they are relatively new. It is believed that nearly all of the mutations occurred in the past 5,000 years, during a time of explosive population growth.

These findings have important implications, the most obvious of which is that there are, indeed, many rare but potent gene mutations present in our genomes that could be responsible for schizophrenia. To identify which ones are pertinent to schizophrenia is another matter, for the statistical problem looms large again. Because the genes are so rare, unrealistically large sample sizes would be required to prove an association between a particular rare gene and schizophrenia. Finally, there is a darker message to be read from these results. As one researcher wrote,

> At least in highly industrialized societies, the impact of deleterious mutations is accumulating on a time scale that is approximately the same as that for scenarios associated with global warming—perhaps not of great concern over a span of one or two generations, but with very considerable consequences on time scales of tens of generations. Without a reduction in the germline [hereditary] transmission of deleterious mutations, the mean phenotypes [physical characteristics] of the residents of industrialized nations are likely to be rather different in just two or three centuries, *with significant incapacitation at the morphological, physiological, and neurobiological levels* [emphasis mine].[13]

Other research points to the need for a fundamental reinterpretation of the data derived from genome-wide association studies, based on the fact (which has been known for many years) that genes constitute less than 2 percent of the total human DNA. Although the remaining 98 percent of DNA is often dismissed as "junk," recent research shows that it has important functions. Rather than containing protein-coding genes, it contains DNA elements that regulate the operation of genes, thereby selectively determining how much protein each gene produces. Remarkably, two recent investigations have discovered that about 90 percent of all single-letter DNA variants occur in these non-protein coding regions of the DNA, that is, in the "junk" rather than in the genes.[14] The implication of this work is that gene variants may be less important than variants found outside of the protein-coding regions. Consequently, variants in the noncoding, regulatory regions are now being studied for possible associations with a variety of diseases including schizophrenia.

Other investigators are focusing on large stretches of protein-coding DNA, some of which include hundreds of individual genes. When cells divide, the DNA in the mother cell is copied to make new DNA for the daughter cells, and errors sometimes occur during the copying process. Sometimes the copying error results in large chunks of DNA being deleted, which means, of course, that some genes will be lost. In other cases, copying errors duplicate portions of DNA, creating in some reported cases as many as 48 separate copies of the same long DNA sequence; this can result in excessive amounts of protein being produced by the affected genes. There is speculation that such variations in gene copy numbers might be linked to diseases; indeed, some studies have reported evidence of an association between copy-number variations and schizophrenia,[15] though others find no such association. So, whether copy-number variation contributes to the risk of schizophrenia remains to be seen.

A dark-horse hypothesis in the whole debate over inheritance of risk comes from a new area of biological research, called **epigenetics**.[16] The focus here is less on DNA than on a special type of protein, called histone protein, which associates with DNA in the cell nucleus. The histone proteins condense the otherwise loose strands of DNA to allow chromosomes to form. It was recently discovered that, in addition to playing this structural role, the histones also play a role in turning genes on and off, hence in regulating the amount of protein made by the genes. The histone-gene interaction can affect protein levels to the same extent as a mutation in the gene itself. And, in the context of schizophrenia, two features of the histones make them particularly relevant. First, the histones' influence on gene activity is regulated by chemical signals coming from outside the cell nucleus, and research has shown that stress is one type of stimulus that can trigger the release of these chemical signals. So, the epigenetic hypothesis incorporates an interaction between genes and the environment, much like the conventional hypothesis based on risk genes. Second, once a gene is turned on or off by a histone protein, it can remain on or off for a lifetime, *and* in some cases the switch can be passed on to the next generation. Chance seems to play a role in whether a given histone switch is inherited in a given generation. As a result, the inheritance of histones is unpredictable, and it therefore mimics the unpredictable inheritance of schizophrenia.

SUMMARY

- Schizophrenia is not caused by any single gene mutation. By comparing the genomes of people who have schizophrenia with those of mentally healthy people, several gene variants that associate with schizophrenia have been identified; these are known as risk genes. However, even if a person has all the known risk genes, he or she will not necessarily develop schizophrenia, and the added risk from having these genes is slight. Clearly, not all sources of genetic risk have yet been identified.

- Most identified risk genes play roles in controlling the development of the brain, from its earliest embryonic stages to adulthood.

- One source of risk for schizophrenia comes from common gene variants. Even though each gene may contribute only a small effect, the combination of large numbers of common gene variants may be crucial. Unfortunately, the DNA from impractically large numbers of individuals will have to be scrutinized to find all the relevant genes.

- Another source of risk lies in a few rare but highly potent mutations. Support for this idea comes from research showing that most gene variants occur in less than 0.5 percent of the population. Again, to identify all the rare mutations will require huge sample sizes.

- When cells divide, they produce an additional copy of their DNA for the new cells. Errors during this process sometimes lead to the deletion or duplication of long sequences of DNA, thus affecting many genes. Some reports claim that variations in copy numbers (deletions or duplications) are associated with schizophrenia.

- According to still another hypothesis, the genes themselves are not altered, but rather their activities are improperly regulated. One source of disruptive regulation lies in the histone proteins, which normally surround the DNA and act as on-off switches for the genes. Another source is the so-called junk DNA, which contains no genes but comprises more than 98 percent of the entire genome; the vast majority of genetic variation is found in this region.

- No matter which genetic agent or agents prove to be responsible, genetic research is essential for improving treatments and possibly preventing schizophrenia.[17]

5

A Consultation with Dr. Held

Although everyone in the family felt the impact of Jim's impending illness, it hit Mom the hardest. She was strong and she was smart, but she never anticipated such a problem. Nor did she find it easy to share her concerns with others. Many years after she died, I was astonished to learn that she rarely spoke of Jim even to her closest friend, a woman with whom she frequently played bridge, shopped, and partied. No, Mom suffered mostly alone, and when Jim's behavior became so troublesome that it demanded a solution, the predicament became hers alone to deal with. Dad was busy with his work as a real estate manager, and he had recently taken on the additional job of teaching at UCLA's Extension. Besides, he was completely out of his element when it came to something like mental illness. In those years, in the United States, no one walked into a medical facility and asked for help with a mentally disturbed son, at least not before the young man got into real trouble. A pervasive stigma blocked the way. Once uncorked, stigma smothered sympathy and inhibited initiative. What, then, was Mom to do, and where could she go for help? Her Jewish background connected her to psychoanalysis, and from there, into the office of Dr. Held.

Psychoanalysis is a therapeutic method based on talking. The ideas behind the method, incorrectly known as the "theory" of psychoanalysis, originated with Sigmund Freud, who worked out the principles in Vienna in the early part of the twentieth century. Although Freud practiced no religion, he was a Jew by ancestry and culture. Most of his professional followers, both in Europe and later in America, were Jewish. Perhaps for this reason, middle-class Jews adopted psychoanalysis with great enthusiasm. According to the historian Edward Shorter, Jews were attracted to psychoanalysis because it allowed them to take pride in an intellectual achievement that was broadly understood to be of revolutionary importance.[1] At a time when the Jews of Central Europe were experiencing the horrors of forced displacements and massive killings, their identification with psychoanalysis provided, in Shorter's words, "a special symbol of self-affirmation, a collective badge of pride." Shorter also points out that psychoanalysis appealed especially to Jewish women; he writes that it was "their thing." My own experience confirms Shorter's views. Although my parents were fully assimilated, second-generation Americans, their identities and their social circles were Jewish, and they felt pride in their intellectual Jewish heroes, like Sigmund Freud and Albert Einstein. Thus, it was only natural that Mom would turn to psychoanalysts for help.

In western Los Angeles, in the late 1950s, psychoanalysis was thriving. Beneath the surface of popular acceptance, however, there were battles raging within the profession itself, conflicts between the European-trained analysts and the American-trained analysts, between the medical analysts and the lay analysts, and between those who adhered to orthodox Freudian methods and those who championed revisionary methods. Much later, I learned that three of the leading players in these disputes were the fathers of Jim's classmates at high school. One father, Dr. Charles Tidd, had been teaching and practicing psychoanalysis in Los Angeles since 1938; he was one of the founding members of the Department of Psychiatry at UCLA. Another father, Dr. Judd Marmor, was a leading psychoanalytic scholar who gained widespread recognition for leading the campaign to remove homosexuality from the professional list of recognized mental illnesses. The third father, Mr. Robert Beasley Jr., was not himself an analyst but was a longtime "lay" member of the board of trustees of the Los Angeles Psychoanalytic Society.

Mom succeeded in getting advice from all three of these individuals. How she managed to do that I do not know, for she was not accustomed to socializing with such people. She was a housewife who spent most of her time with domestic chores and in outings with women friends. Most of Mom and Dad's friends were middle-class business people.

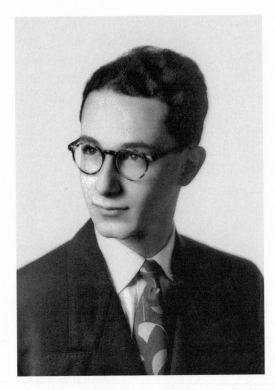

**Jim's high school
graduation portrait,
1952**

I can only imagine how my mother might have approached the analysts.
She probably used the phone in her bedroom, at night behind a closed
door.

"Hello, Dr. Tidd, my name is Ruth Chase. My son and your son were
classmates at University High School. I am so sorry to bother you, but I
hope that you can spare a few minutes to talk to me."

"Well, yes, I suppose so. What's your son's name?"

"Jim, or James. He's a tall, lanky fellow, and a good student. He's a
graduate student at UCLA now. He started out in chemistry, but he
switched to English. He likes to read."

"I don't know him."

"Where should I begin?" asked Mom, but she did not wait for an answer. "It's about Jim. He's changed recently, and he's become very difficult to deal with. I know there is something bothering him, but he won't

tell me what it is. In fact, he doesn't speak much to anyone anymore. He spends a lot of time in his room with the door shut. I'm afraid of what he might be doing in there. And then, there are the unpredictable, violent outbursts. We may be enjoying a meal together—with my husband and a younger son—when Jim will suddenly shout out obscenities and throw food or other objects. He nearly hurt Ronnie the other day when he threw a plate at him. And yet, at other times, he and Ronnie get along quite well together."

"Oh, I see," said Dr. Tidd. "And does Jim have friends at school or elsewhere?"

"He has two friends from school. Both are quiet types like Jim, and one comes to our house occasionally. Or at least he did up until a few months ago."

Dr. Tidd pressed the inquiry. "What about girls? Does he have a girlfriend?"

"No," Mom replied. "And he doesn't talk on the phone with girls either . . . not as far as I can tell anyway. His younger brother is constantly on the phone with girls."

"Well, Mrs. Chase, from what you've told me, it would appear that your son is stressed from the demands of his studies at UCLA. If he is a serious student, as you say he is, then the heavy workload is probably affecting his social life. This type of reaction is not unusual. Many young men find it difficult to transition from high school to university."

"No, no," Mom insisted. "It's more than that, I am sure it's more. Jim is very intelligent, so I can't imagine that his coursework could be so difficult. And besides, what about the shouting and the violent behavior? No, Dr. Tidd, I'm very worried. Jim was such a sweet boy when he was younger, but he has recently become a different person, someone whom I hardly know. It hurts me to say this, but it is the truth."

She was on the verge of tears. In a voice full of desperation she appealed directly to the doctor, "Please, Dr. Tidd, you've got to help me. I think there is something very wrong with my son."

"Yes, of course, I understand," replied Dr. Tidd. "I was only giving you an impression based on what you had said. It was not my professional judgment. I would never give you a diagnosis over the phone without first seeing your son. Unfortunately, I am not able to see him at this time. My schedule at UCLA does not permit me to take more private patients."

"Oh, I'm sorry to hear that. I was so hoping that you could help me."

"There are many other excellent psychoanalysts . . . let me think . . . I believe Dr. Albert Held would be appropriate. He's a skilled therapist with a well-established practice in Beverly Hills. I can also vouch for the orthodoxy of his training in psychoanalysis. He has a good grasp of theory. I suggest you give him a call, and when you do, please mention that I recommended him."

Dr. Tidd had his facts right when he referred to the abundance of psychoanalysts in Los Angeles. The historian Edward Shorter notes the steadily rising influence of psychoanalysis in America in the period from the end of World War II to the mid-1960s. He cites surveys that showed that "by 1966, a third of American psychiatrists had received some kind of psychoanalytic training, and 67 percent said that they employed 'the dynamic approach' [the psychoanalytic approach] with their patients. By the mid-1960s, psychiatry had come in the mind of the American public to mean psychoanalysis." Shorter goes on to say, "The most baleful aspect of the takeover of psychiatry by psychoanalysts was the analysts' ambition to extend their theories to the diagnosis and treatment of psychotic illness."[2] An ill-conceived theory has a greater potential to cause harm when applied to psychotic illnesses compared to the milder "neurotic" illnesses.

The leading authority on the psychoanalytic treatment of psychotic illnesses was Dr. Frieda Fromm-Reichmann, a German contemporary of Freud's who immigrated to the United States during World War II. She wrote that psychoanalysis could help a person who had schizophrenia

> if he was approached by a psychiatrist who knew that the patient's longing for interpersonal contact was just as intense as his fear of it, which had originally driven him into a state of regression and withdrawal. That is, an intensively charged relationship could be established between the schizophrenic patient and the psychiatrist.[3]

She went on to make the following infamous statement:

> The schizophrenic is painfully distrustful and resentful of other people, due to the severe early warp and rejection he encountered in important people of his infancy and childhood, as a rule, *mainly in a schizophrenogenic mother* [emphasis mine].[4]

Yes, you read correctly. My mother had managed to deliver herself into the hands of a doctor who believed that schizophrenia was caused by a "schizophrenogenic mother," or at least I assume that this was the case, because Albert Held was a psychoanalyst, analysts generally followed the advice of a few prominent leaders, and Frieda Fromm-Reichmann was one of those leaders. I cannot say for certain that Dr. Held shared Dr. Fromm-Reichmann's views on schizophrenia, but there is little doubt that most psychiatrists, including most psychoanalysts, accepted her ideas about psychosis. One scholar has said of this period that it had become "standard practice to believe that mothers were the cause of their children's psychosis."[5] It does not take much imagination to comprehend the effect on Mom.

Although it had been happening for some time, I was slow to notice that Dad and Jim left the house together every Tuesday and Thursday afternoon. They took the car, and they returned an hour and a half later. When I finally asked where they had gone, Mom said that Jim was visiting an immunologist to determine the source of his allergies. Several weeks later, however, I learned the true purpose of these trips when Mom announced that she, Dad, and I would be seeing Dr. Held in his Beverly Hills office. The time had come to learn what was bothering Jim. So we drove the short distance to Beverly Hills and parked the car on North Bedford Drive. The street was filled with jewelry stores and upscale clothing establishments. At a small medical building we proceeded upstairs to the doctor's office.

"Please, make yourselves comfortable," said Dr. Held, as he gestured toward the three empty chairs arranged in front of his desk. The late afternoon sun cast soft shadows as it filtered through the white curtains behind us. I noticed a half-open door into an adjacent room and guessed that it was in there that Dr. Held listened to his patients. After exchanging pleasantries, Dr. Held got to the heart of the matter.

"I must confess," he began, "Jim's case is difficult. As you know, Jim is highly intelligent. He has a good memory and the ability to reason logically. As well, I don't mind telling you, I find him very interesting as a patient. However, as you are surely aware, some aspects of his psyche are unbalanced and in need of repair. Naturally, I cannot recount for you the details of our therapeutic sessions nor explain at any length my evaluation of his psychodynamics. Those things must remain confidential. What I can say is that Jim suffers from recurring fears and anxieties. Sometimes he hears internal voices, and many of his ideas are bizarre, to say the least. He keeps most of this to himself because he believes that others will not understand him and, importantly, he himself cannot distinguish the valid ideas from those that are pure fantasy. With so much going on inside his head, he has largely withdrawn from the external world. As a result, he is having difficulties in his relationships and in coping with the demands of everyday life. He is lonely and, I must say, quite desperate."

"Yes, but these things we already know," said Mom. "We were hoping that you would tell us what the future holds for Jim. Can you help him? Can you free him of these problems? When will he be okay again?"

Dr. Held was smoking one cigarette after another. Whenever he finished a cigarette, he crushed the butt into a small glass ashtray on top of his well-polished wooden desk. At this point in the consultation, the ashtray became full. As we were waiting for him to reply to Mom's prodding, he reached down, opened a side drawer of the desk, and swiftly dumped the contents of the ashtray into a hidden receptacle. Equally quickly, he shut the drawer and returned the ashtray to the desk. It was as though he had buried Jim's troubles in that drawer.

"It is difficult to say how long it will take, Mrs. Chase. Jim needs a thorough psychoanalysis and, unfortunately, the process cannot be rushed. Although we have just begun to explore his unconscious dynamics, I have noted a partial emotional regression. He is motivated by a fear of repetitional rejection, a distrust of others, and his own retaliative hostility. Oh, I'm sorry. I lapsed into jargon. All I wish to say is that we are discovering that Jim's mind is filled with imaginative but false ideas. He and I have a lot of work to do to find the psychodynamic roots of these delusions. Only then will he feel better. The entire process will require months, if not years. And, to be completely honest with you, I cannot guarantee that we will be successful."

Dad spoke up for the first time. "What do you mean, it may not be successful?"

"I mean that no matter what we do here, or for how long, I may not be able to help him. He may get worse. I cannot predict the outcome."

Dr. Held stopped speaking, and he seemed to hold his breath as he stared at us, eyes bulging with frustration. Mom's face had suddenly grown long and tired. I, too, was taken down by what I had heard. Although Dad was clearly angry, he sat sternly and said nothing more. He refused to accept that a man of Dr. Held's reputation, a man who commanded exorbitant fees for his work, could not fix my brother's problems. Many years later—in fact, shortly before his death—Jim related to me an exchange that he had overheard between Dad and an unnamed psychiatrist. I didn't ask whether it was Dr. Held, but it might have been. Evidently, the doctor had been spouting a bunch of psychiatric hogwash. Jim proudly recalled Dad's words in replying to the doctor, "I don't give a damn about all your fancy theories! I just want you to make my son better!" At this meeting with Dr. Held, however, there was nothing more for any of us to say.

Dr. Held took a final puff on his cigarette, crushed it in the ashtray, and opened the desk drawer. Once again, I stared in amazement as he deftly disposed of the butts. We thanked the doctor, he wished us well, and we shook hands before leaving his office. Jim's sessions with Dr. Held continued for another year or so—up until, but not after, his initial psychotic crisis.

6

Which Aspects of the Environment
Cause Schizophrenia?

I have said that 80 percent of the risk for schizophrenia is due to genes, with the remaining risk due to the environment. I also mentioned that a person with the same genes as a person with schizophrenia– that is, an identical twin–has about an even chance of getting schizophrenia or avoiding it. These facts (discussed in chapter 4) strongly suggest that a person's early experiences play a role in determining whether he or she develops schizophrenia.

Some scientists look upon the genes as establishing the liability, while the environment provides the trigger. The genetic risk factors and the environmental risk factors might be independent variables that add to one another to create a total risk. Alternatively, according to the more nuanced view held by many scientists, the genes and the environment interact so that the effects of each variable (genes, the environment) depend on the other variable. An example of interaction would be where a gene mutation increases a person's sensitivity to an environmental stimulus, say a virus: when the person encounters the virus, the person's heightened sensitivity allows an infection in the brain; the infection disrupts normal brain development, which causes mental illness. Regardless of whether one sees the genetic and environmental contributions as additive or interactive, some combination of both elements is required to produce schizophrenia.[1]

Epidemiologists define the environment as the entire surroundings in which a person lives, including its physical, social, and cultural aspects. Understood from the perspective of a growing child or adolescent, "the environment" represents every thing and every event that impacts on his or her physical and psychological development. Clearly, myriad factors need to be considered in searching for the key environmental determinants of schizophrenia. The task is made especially difficult by the fact that schizophrenia typically becomes manifest only in late adolescence or early adulthood, which means that many years of experience must be reviewed for relevant evidence.[2]

Early investigators focused on events and experiences that are highly stressful. They were surprised to learn that neither war combat nor the divorce of one's parents precipitates schizophrenia. On the other hand, schizophrenia does associate rather strongly with urban environments and migration, both of which can be seen as stressful, though less stressful than war and divorce. Why, then, are these less stressful environments more closely tied to schizophrenia than the more stressful ones? I mentioned one possibility earlier—namely, that city living and migration are proxies for other factors that simply accompany city living and migration, for example, exposure to infections. It is also possible that there is something about people with schizophrenia, or people at risk for schizophrenia, that causes them to go to cities or move to a new country. Stress, therefore, may be irrelevant to the associations of schizophrenia with urban living and migration. Pending further research, we are left to conclude that while stress *might* cause schizophrenia, it cannot be proved by a statistical correlation between a particular type of environment, which happens to be stressful, and schizophrenia. Unfortunately, people—scientists included—too often mistake evidence of correlation (association) for evidence of causation.

Among the other nongenetic factors that appear to be associated with schizophrenia are the father's age at the time of his child's birth and marijuana (cannabis) use. The effect of the father's age, though rather small, is well supported by data. It is probably explained by the fact that mutations in sperm cells increase with increasing age. On average, a 20-year-old father passes on about 20 mutations to his child, whereas a 40-year-old father transmits about 65 mutations.[3] The effect of marijuana use is also well supported by relevant studies, and it entails an even larger risk.[4] One study in Sweden followed more than 45,000 army conscripts. Fifteen years after conscription, the men who had smoked marijuana had more than twice the rate of schizophrenia as those who had not smoked marijuana. At 27 years out, there was a threefold difference between users and non-users. The younger the age when marijuana use begins, the greater the risk of psychosis. Also, the risk increases with increased frequency of use and with highly potent marijuana. In the Swedish study, "heavy users" were six times more likely to get schizophrenia than non-users.

Much attention has been directed toward events very early in life, because this is when the brain experiences its most rapid growth. A disruption in the normal program of brain development is thought to lay the foundation for the later appearance of schizophrenia. (The science of brain development is discussed in chapter 8.) A considerable amount of evidence points to critical events around the time of birthing. Obstetric complications constitute one category of factors, including fetal hypoxia (low oxygen), small birth weight, small head size, and emergency caesarean section. When the birthing mother has diabetes, the child is nearly eight times more likely to develop schizophrenia than when the mother has no diabetes, even when mothers are matched for sex of the child, age of the mother, social class, and hospital of birth. Schizophrenia has also been linked to the mother's inadequate nutrition, especially foliate deficiency and vitamin D deficiency.

One of the more controversial areas of research concerns the role of maternal infections. Early studies indicated that infants born in the winter months were more likely to develop schizophrenia as adults than infants born at other times. (Jim was born on December 30.) Although these studies were later criticized for design flaws and inconsistent results, investigators were intrigued by the idea that the winter months might have exposed either the fetus or the infant to infections. Other studies, which were also contentious, reported an increased **incidence** of schizophrenia among individuals who were growing in the womb during influenza epidemics. Far from controversial, on the other hand, is the fact that certain bacteria, viruses, and other infectious agents are capable of causing congenital brain anomalies that lead to behavioral disorders.

With all of this as background, several recent studies have reexamined the link between infections and schizophrenia. These new studies used a so-called **prospective** design in which investigators began by identifying mothers who were known to have had an infection during pregnancy. The offspring of those pregnancies were then tracked down as adults to learn how many of them had developed schizophrenia, and the results were compared with another group of offspring born of mothers who had not been infected but who were otherwise similar to the first group in age, socioeconomic status, location, and so on. The results were significant: the risk of schizophrenia increased five times with rubella infections; five times with maternal genital or reproductive infections; either seven times or three times with influenza infections, depending on whether the infection occurred early (seven times) or late (three times) in pregnancy; and two times for infections of the single-cell parasite *Toxoplasma gondii*.[5]

Another area of obvious concern in the child's life is the psychological and social environment. Psychoanalysis was originally founded on the notion that early family interactions are central to understanding the genesis of psychiatric conditions. Frieda Fromm-Reichmann's invention of the schizophrenogenic mother (mentioned in chapter 5) gradually morphed into the idea of the schizophrenogenic family; in this portrayal, how emotions are expressed and how the child and his or her parents communicate are assumed to be the main factors leading to psychosis. There have been numerous variations on this theme. Summing up the opinions of experts in 1974, one psychiatrist wrote in the *American Journal of Psychiatry*:

> From the first period of life the future schizophrenic finds himself in a family that is not able to offer him a modicum of security or basic trust. The world he meets in childhood consists of interpersonal relations characterized by intense anxiety or hostility, by false detachment, or by a combination of these feelings. Some authors have attributed great psychogenetic importance to the abnormality of the family as a whole; others have focused on the unhappy marriage of the parents or on the personality of the father or on the interaction with the siblings. The personality and attitude of the mother remain, in the opinion of many, the most important psychogenic factors.[6]

Clearly, many psychiatrists believed, in 1974, that family dynamics cause schizophrenia. Nevertheless, the evidence for such a conclusion was, in fact, weak at that time because almost all the relevant information was obtained from interviews with patients. That is, the patients told the investigators about their families, and the investigators drew conclusions. Apart from the bias inherent in sourcing the information from the patient, there is also the problem of knowing whether the reported family situation is the *cause* of the mental illness or the *result* of the illness. One can readily imagine, for example, that a family might became nonfunctional *because* of the patient's illness. Once again, the way to resolve such ambiguities is to conduct a prospective study in which families are first assessed by an unbiased, professional investigator before there is any obvious mental illness and then followed up later to determine in which families, if any, children developed psychoses. Even now, there have been surprisingly few such studies.

One prospective study, reported in 1987, looked at 64 families, each of which contained a teenager who was considered to be "disturbed" but not clinically ill.[7] The families were interviewed intensively to obtain information on how family members communicated with each other. Afterward, several predefined aspects of communication were rated using a numerical scale. The investigators returned to the families 5 and 15 years later to find out what had become of the previously "disturbed" teenagers, now young adults. They found that schizophrenia and schizophrenia-like disorders were most likely to develop in those children whose parents were rated low on their ability to maintain attention when speaking to another person and high on their use of critical and hostile communications. A third measure, the amount of emotional expression in the parents' communications, had no effect on the children's outcomes.

The positive results from this study are statistically significant, and they should be considered together with the adoption study mentioned in chapter 4, which found that adopted children who inherit a genetic risk are more likely to develop schizophrenia if they grow up in a dysfunctional family rather than in a "healthy" family. And, growing up in a family in which either a parent or a sibling has schizophrenia is clearly not sufficient to cause schizophrenia in the absence of a genetic liability, that is, when the parent or sibling belongs to the adopting family. Confusing though these scenarios may be, they tell us that the family environment interacts with the genetic endowment. Certain types of family environments, such as those with strained communications, can precipitate schizophrenia in individuals who carry a genetic liability, whereas well-functioning family environments can protect at-risk individuals from developing schizophrenia.

The special case of identical twins brings into focus some questions about how the family environment shapes child development. Ordinarily, two identical twins will share not just the same genes but also the same family environment, at least during their early formative years. So, how do we explain one identical twin getting schizophrenia while the other twin does not? Asking this question prompts us to ask the more general question, Why do *any* two siblings grow up to be different? After all, even non-twin pairs have 50 percent of their genes in common (on average), and they share the same family environment. Is it the difference in the genes or the difference in the family environment that makes siblings different?

Some compelling research has led to a remarkable conclusion: once genetic relatedness is taken into account, two children growing up in the same household are no more similar to each other than any two kids chosen at random and growing up in separate households.[8] These findings suggest that children raised together in the same family have quite different experiences. In fact, according to in-depth studies of family interactions, the experiences of two siblings living in the same household are as different as those of any two children chosen at random from the general population.

Social scientists wanted to know which specific aspects of the family environment are experienced differently by two children in the same household. They discounted such factors as economic status and quality of the parents' marriage because it was assumed that these things would affect all children similarly. Instead, they focused on such factors as the parents being more affectionate toward one child than the other, and the relationships between the siblings themselves. Also considered were family structure factors such as the order of births and the age differences between the children.

Most of the studies examined the effects of these differences on adolescent personalities and **cognitive** abilities. Drs. Eric Turkheimer and

Mary Waldron, from the University of Virginia, rigorously analyzing the data from 43 studies of the type described, came to a disappointing conclusion.[9] When genetic influences were controlled for, the cumulative effect of all specifically defined environmental factors accounted for less than 2 percent of the differences. The remaining 98 percent of the environmental influence was attributed to undefined (unknown) factors. Clearly, social scientists still have much to learn about how the family environment affects childhood psychological development. It also follows that psychiatrists cannot yet identify which aspects of the family environment trigger schizophrenic illness in children who carry a genetic risk for the disease.

As research advances and we learn more about the genetic and environmental factors associated with schizophrenia, it may become possible to predict who is likely to develop schizophrenia. Alternatively, some investigators are currently trying to make predictions based not on genetics or the environment but on observations of the child. The best of these studies are prospective in design and use formal tests to measure various behavioral and psychological characteristics.[10] They find that low intelligence and delayed or incomplete motor skills are the strongest predictors of later schizophrenia; although the associations are quite small, they are nonetheless statistically significant.

It is important to note that no amount of direct observation or formal testing is sufficient to predict whether a young child will develop schizophrenia, even when such data are combined with genetic information and brain scans. Most children with low intelligence or poor motor skills *do not* develop schizophrenia. Not until around age 18 can a future psychotic breakdown be predicted with any certainty, and only then if the individual has a close relative with schizophrenia *and* is already showing behavioral or psychological signs of disturbance.[11] Finally, no indicator of future schizophrenia should be confused with causation. Although certain behaviors in animals are said to predict earthquakes, no one would argue that animals cause earthquakes.

SUMMARY

- Schizophrenia is caused partly by genes and partly by the environment, where the latter term refers to the totality of an individual's experiences. Neither the responsible genes nor the responsible aspects of the environment have yet been identified. There are probably many specific causes, both genetic and environmental, with different combinations determining illness in different people.

- The environmental risks and the genetic risks may simply add to one another; or, alternatively, the environmental effects may depend on the nature of the genetic risks. Regardless, most authorities believe that the genes establish a liability, and the environment delivers a trigger.

- The early environment is thought to be especially important. The factors most highly correlated with later schizophrenia are obstetric complications, maternal infections, maternal dietary deficiencies, and minor congenital abnormalities. Older fathers are associated with greater risk, probably because the likelihood of spermatic gene mutations increases with age. Also, the use of marijuana increases risk, especially when begun at a young age and when involving highly potent varieties of marijuana.

- Although family interactions are widely thought to be important, research has yet to identify the specific aspects of these interactions that affect the development of schizophrenia.

7

Breakdown in Westwood Village

The spring of 1958 was, for some, a joyous time. The economy was strong, the American spirit was swollen with confidence, and the magnolia tree in our front yard was in full bloom; we loved the tree's sweet-smelling, cream-colored flowers. Also, many of our friends were excited because the Brooklyn Dodgers baseball team had just become the Los Angeles Dodgers. In our house, though, there was little to cheer about.

My brother was taking graduate-level courses in English literature at UCLA, and he had recently moved into a small apartment on Gayley Avenue close by the campus. The university was of a modest size in those days, and the adjacent commercial district, still known today as West-wood Village, was fully deserving of its quaint moniker. Jim could have walked to the campus from our house, but considering the state of tension that had developed in our home, Mom and Dad thought that it would be in his best interest, and ours, if he were to have his own apartment. The room that they rented for him was on a busy street near several fraternity houses. It was from this room that Jim phoned home to announce that he was about to kill first his girlfriend and then himself.

Actually, it was not really an announcement but an anguished cry for help. Why else would he bother to call? I was using the phone extension in my room to eavesdrop on the conversation when I heard Mom's pleading, "Jimmy! Jimmy! Please! Calm down. We can help you. You'll be okay."

"The hell I will. I'm going to use the gun."

Mom tried a different tactic, "What is the girl's name? She must be very nice. Where did you meet her?"

"*Oh shut up*! You don't know a goddamn thing about anything!" Clearly, Mom's tactic was not succeeding.

"Jim, this is Dad. What is the problem? Just tell me what the problem is. We can help you."

After several long seconds waiting for Jim to reply, the silence was broken by a click and then a steady ring tone. Jim had hung up. I moved to the door of my bedroom, surreptitiously opened it a bit more, and positioned myself so I could listen without being seen to listen. Mom was completely beside herself. Between sobs she shouted at Dad, "Do something! Do something! Don't just stand there, do something!"

"What *can* we do?" Dad replied in a pleading sort of way.

"You can call Dr. Held. Quick, call him. Oh, hell, I'll do it myself." Mom dialed several times before she was able to speak with Dr. Held.

"Hello, this is Mrs. Chase, Jim's mother. I'm sorry to disturb you, but we are very worried about Jim. He phoned us from his apartment, saying that he has a gun. He's threatening to use it. There's a girl with him too—or at least she was there was a few minutes ago—we're afraid he might harm her. We tried to calm him down, but he hung up on us. Please, please help us! I want you to phone him and talk to him. Will you do that?"

Dr. Held did phone Jim, and he did speak briefly with him, on two occasions. Each time, Jim listened but said little. After a few minutes on both calls, Jim hung up the receiver.

"Hello Mrs. Chase, this is Dr. Held. I spoke to Jim. He is certainly angry and very disturbed. There are many ideas running through his mind, and I am afraid that he is losing touch with reality. Unfortunately, he is not relating to me in a rational manner, so there is little that I can do right now. I can only suggest that you call the police."

Mom did not want to call the police, at least not yet. To do so would be to acknowledge the seriousness of the situation. She dreaded the idea of Jim being dragged away in handcuffs or, worse, tossed into a jail cell. Nevertheless, the gun weighed heavily on her mind. Jim had threatened to use it. Would he? Violence was not in his nature, and yet he was changing into a person she no longer knew. Maybe Jim was feeling better now; maybe he had calmed down. She decided to phone him. I went to my room and picked up the phone extension.

"Hello, Jimmy dear."

Silence. And then, "Leave me alone."

"Are you feeling better dear?"

"What do you care how I am feeling? You're just saying that. I'll tell you who cares about me—no one cares! Even I don't care anymore. Mother, I'm telling you, even after I'm dead and gone, no one will care. It just doesn't matter."

"What about the girl?" Mom asked. "What did you say her name was?"

"Bitch, that's her name. She's gone. Now it's just me and my gun. I'm ready to go too. The next time you call, there won't be anyone here to answer the phone. I'll be dead and gone."

"Jimmy, Jimmy, we love you. Stop talking to me like that. Please, we are coming to see you."

"You'd better not!" Then, *click*, and the ring tone sounded; he had hung up.

Meanwhile, Dad speeded on his way over to Jim's place in his car. When he knocked on the door, there was no answer. He knocked again, and Jim shouted back at him, "*Go away! I don't want to talk to you!*" Dad pleaded with Jim to open the door, but he only managed to provoke further insults. Finally, Dad returned home with his heart full of fear.

By the time Dad got back, I was out of my bedroom. Mom told me what had been happening, but I already knew more than she suspected. She was calmer now, starting to get control of herself and take charge. Her change of behavior calmed me down as well. The three of us—Mom, Dad, and I—gathered in the living room to discuss the situation. Before long, Mom decided on a course of action, and soon Dad was on the phone speaking with a supervisor at the local police station.

"No, we've tried that," he said. "We also reached his psychiatrist, who told us that he can't help us. He was the one who suggested that we phone the police. Really, we have no other options. Please, you must hurry. Here is the address. . . . What? What do you mean you can't *do* anything!" Dad argued with the supervisor for several minutes before he slammed down the phone in disgust.

"He told me that the police will only intervene if there is violence or if violence is imminent. They are not allowed to arrest someone just because he is acting irrationally. And, since the girl is no longer in the apartment, the only person that Jim might harm is himself. I felt like telling him to go to hell! But he was adamant. Unless the situation changes, there is nothing that they can do."

Each of us then fell silent, tormented by horrible thoughts. Mom was so consumed with fear and frustration that she began to cry. However, she quickly wiped away the tears and focused on regaining her strength. She lifted up the telephone and dialed Jim's apartment number. She let the phone ring for a minute or so, but there was no answer. Not knowing what to do next, we sat silently until . . . *our* telephone rang. As soon as Dad picked up the receiver, I went into my room to listen in.

"I'm finished," said Jim.

"What do you mean 'finished'?" Dad asked. "Are you okay?"

"I'm finished with everything. I need to leave here. Can you pick me up? I want to go home."

"Sure, I'll come right over. Are you okay? Is the girl—I don't know her name—is she okay?"

"I told you, she left. I didn't use the gun."

Jim came home still agitated and confused. He said very little to any of us, went into his room, and stayed there for the better part of two weeks. We heard him shout obscenities from behind his closed door, and we endured further unpleasant scenes at the dinner table. We asked Jim what was troubling him, but he did not tell us; he likely did not know himself. Although no one spoke about psychosis or schizophrenia, we realized the seriousness of the situation. Painfully aware of our inability to help Jim, Mom suggested to him that he might want to seek treatment in a hospital. Fortunately, Jim remained rational enough to see possibilities in this idea, and a few days later, he announced that he was prepared to sign in at a nearby psychiatric hospital.

Jim was now 24 years old. He would never again live with his family. Instead, during the next 41 years, he resided in 14 hospitals (8 psychiatric, 6 medical); 5 board-and-care facilities; 1 halfway house; and 5 apartment buildings (short stays only).

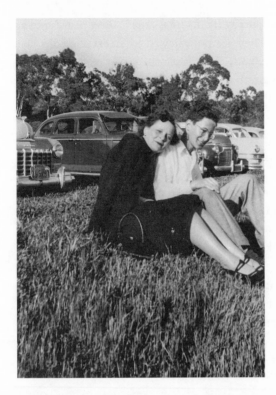

**Jim and his mother at
Will Rogers State Park,
1957**

The first of the hospitals, the Crestwood, was privately operated, very small, and located on a Los Angeles street bustling with shops and businesses. A formidable fence covered in dark ivy protected the premises from the street view, and the doorway was shaded by the fronds of a large palm tree. No sign identified the building as a hospital. Inside, a lobby led off to rooms at the back where the patients resided and where "services" were rendered. Its limited capacity, unusual location, and high cost meant that patients did not remain there long. Jim, in fact, moved to another hospital after a two-week stay.

His next stop was the Edgemont Hospital, newly opened and located in the heart of Hollywood. It, too, was a private facility, and even more expensive than the Crestwood. We soon saw what money can buy when Mom, Dad, and I went to visit Jim. Dad drove east along Hollywood Boulevard until he came to a marked lane bordered on either side by Lombardy poplars. He turned into the lane and headed up a gentle slope to reach the hospital, which sat perched on a hilly prominence. He parked the car nearby. Then we steeled ourselves for what was to come and walked into the reception building. Inside, the newly upholstered furniture, the serene oil paintings, and the polished surfaces were all shimmering in warm light. It was as if we were being welcomed at the reception desk of a comfortable European hotel. Or perhaps a summer camp, for Jim was living with several other patients in a kind of cottage on a grassy knoll behind and below the reception building. It was there that we found him, just two days after his initial treatment with electroconvulsive shock.

As my brother's life later unfolded, the short stays at Crestwood Hospital and Edgemont Hospital would be remembered for the mixed feelings of hope and dread. We wanted to believe that the professionalism that was so much on display at Edgemont would make Jim well again. Electroconvulsive shock seemed an extreme measure, but if that was what Jim needed, then we were ready to accept it. Jim, however, saw things differently, and he had the better view. A few years after he left Edgemont Hospital, he wrote about his stay there. In the following excerpt, he recalls his thoughts as Dad drove him back to the hospital after an evening at the family home in Westwood.

> Moving through this glitter, this life, I felt hopeless; it seemed to me that I would never have a woman myself, that I would spend the remainder of my life in the hospital, in the dullness and monotony, with only rare respites such as this night when I would go into the town with my father. The future was a bleak desert, and I felt rebellion rise within me. I would have liked to take my fate and strangle it, but it had me in a helpless grip. . . . I asked my father how long he thought I was going to remain in the hospital. He said he thought I could get out very soon, that he expected improvement at any moment, that I had every cause to be optimistic. He asked what I thought, and I answered I expected to be in the hospital for the rest of my life. He protested, said I should not take that attitude, said that all the signs pointed to my getting well. . . . I made no reply. I wanted to let him have his faith, even though I knew differently.

8

Why Does Schizophrenia Begin
in Late Adolescence?

Adolescence brings changes to body, mind, and behavior. Although we do not ordinarily associate adolescence with the onset of disease and ill health, the major mental illnesses, including schizophrenia, depression, and bipolar disease, all emerge during adolescence. Diagnoses of schizophrenia peak in the late teen years and the early twenties for men, and a few years later, around age 25 years, for women. These ages refer to the adult-onset type of schizophrenia. An early-onset type of schizophrenia (childhood schizophrenia) typically begins between the ages of 5 and 10 years, but it is about 100 times less common than the adult-onset type.

In contrast to the so-called mental diseases, other diseases of the nervous system tend to appear either very early in life (cerebral palsy, mental retardation) or very late in life (Parkinson's, Alzheimer's, and other dementias). Exceptionally, a few neurological disorders can begin *either* early in life *or* late in life, and their behavioral and psychological symptoms vary depending on the age of onset. One such disorder is Huntington's disease, which caught the attention of Daniel Weinberger, then chief scientist at the Clinical Brain Disorders Branch of the U.S. National Institute of Mental Health. Weinberger first noted that while the microscopic signs of nerve cell degeneration in Huntington's disease are very similar regardless of the age of onset, the psychiatric features, in contrast, can be quite different depending on when the disease begins.[1] In children, psychological symptoms of any kind are rare; in adolescence, schizophrenia-like symptoms occur; in adult years, depression occurs; and in senior years, dementia is most likely.

By studying the clinical facts concerning Huntington's disease and other diseases with variable times of onset, Weinberger reached the conclusion that the adolescent brain is especially susceptible to mental disturbances. In a highly influential article published in 1987, he proposed that schizophrenia originates very early in life as the brain begins to grow. He went on to describe the "critical phase" of brain development that occurs during adolescence, and he suggested that schizophrenia becomes apparent in late adolescence or early adulthood because that is when the brain is challenged to meet new functional demands. In his words, "Schizophrenia is a **neurodevelopmental** disorder in which a fixed brain lesion [structural defect] from early in life interacts with certain normal maturational events that occur much later. The thesis rests on the clinical maxim that the manifestations of a brain lesion vary with the state of brain maturation." Although now widely accepted by psychiatric experts, the characterization of schizophrenia as a disorder of nervous system development remains a scientific hypothesis. Much of the available evidence is consistent with the hypothesis, but none proves it conclusively. And, as I will explain below, several different versions of the hypothesis vie for our attention.

The neurodevelopmental perspective on schizophrenia arises from the incredible complexity of the human brain; indeed, the human brain is one of the most complex objects in the entire universe. Its extraordinary capabilities are made possible by the coordinated actions of about one trillion nerve cells, or **neurons**. Thoughts and actions arise when groups of neurons "talk" to one another using both electrical and chemical signals. To work properly, the communication circuits within the brain must be built according to a fairly specific structural plan, a plan that evolved over millions of years. If the circuits are not constructed according to this plan, problems quickly arise. As a simple example, if neuron A is meant to connect to neuron B but is instead connected to neuron C, then the message that A sends to C will be misinterpreted because it was supposed to go to B. Multiply an error like that by many millions of equivalent A, B, and C neurons, and a thought can go horribly wrong. To build the brain correctly is an intricate task demanding unimaginable precision.

Normal development of the human brain begins in the fetus and ends almost three decades later. It starts with the production of neurons and support cells (glia cells), at the rate of approximately 50,000 new cells *every second*. Each neuron must then migrate from the place of its birth to its predetermined anatomical position, from which point it extends a long, thin structure known as the **axon**. Electrical impulses will later travel down the length of the axon to be passed on to recipient cells. Thus, it is crucially important that the axons extend in the correct direction *and* that they connect with the right target neurons.

How is all of this accomplished? The process is governed by molecules (mostly proteins) that are produced from genetic blueprints. One comprehensive investigation found that at least 15,132 genes, or 86.1 percent of all genes in the human genome, are active during development of the brain. This is a remarkable finding. The molecules that are produced by these genes control many aspects of neural development. They regulate the conversion of precursor cells to nerve cells, they establish chemical gradients that guide growing axons, and they create unique chemical signatures on cell membranes that allow the axon terminals to recognize appropriate targets. Each gene is turned on and off in sequence according to a predetermined timetable, so that the proteins required for each task will be present at the right time and in the right place. With errors in early brain development identified as the likely starting point for schizophrenia, and with gene actions so important for building the brain, it figures that faulty genes would be implicated as causes of the disease.

The vulnerable nature of brain development brings into focus the studies, reviewed in the previous chapter, that connect specific aspects of a child's early environment with the probability that he or she will later develop schizophrenia. Inadequate maternal nutrition, maternal infections, and difficulties at delivery are statistically associated with schizophrenia, and each of these factors can also interfere with normal brain development. The fact remains, however, that most children who later develop schizophrenia appear normal until late adolescence.[2] This raises the question, if schizophrenia is caused by a problem during early brain development, why does it not become manifest until late adolescence? One way to answer this question is to look at some of the major events of adolescence, especially as they relate to the brain.

Adolescence is a period when major physical, emotional, and social changes take place. Cognitive functions are sharpened at this time, and behavioral skills mature. These events are driven by changes in the levels of circulating hormones. Some of the hormones enter the brain, where they bring about anatomical changes, notably in the cerebral **cortex**. Researchers use imaging methods such as magnetic resonance imaging (MRI) to monitor the structural changes that occur over the course of several years in individual brains. With variations in the technique, it is possible to look separately at the *gray matter*, which comprises areas of the brain that are rich in neuronal cell bodies and **dendrites**, and the *white matter*, which comprises the fibrous tracts that run between various regions. The fibers are, in fact, aggregates of neuronal axons. They appear white because each axon is wrapped in a fatty blanket composed of myelin. From such studies, it is known that the total volume of gray matter declines during normal adolescence, while the volume of white matter increases in the same period. Together, these results imply that the brain is partially restructured during adolescence. It is significant, therefore, that the brains of people who have schizophrenia show a significantly greater reduction of gray matter than do the brains of healthy individuals. Moreover, much of the white matter has an abnormal physical appearance in brains of people who have schizophrenia.[3]

Other studies investigate the brains of people who die at various ages, that is, they examine brains postmortem. Significant changes are again seen around the time of adolescence. Most striking is the reduction in the number of synapses. This finding is consistent with the decline in gray matter, because synapses are usually located on dendrites, the structures that fill the gray matter. The loss of synapses is interpreted as a sign of *pruning*, whereby ineffectual and inappropriate neuronal connections are eliminated during the adolescent years to make room for more useful ones. Synapses play a critical role in information processing, so errors made during pruning have the potential to cause serious problems.

The changes I have described are seen in all regions of the normal adolescent cerebral cortex, but the changes affecting the frontal lobe merit special attention because of the unique functions of this lobe and its likely involvement in schizophrenia. Part of the frontal lobe, known as the **prefrontal cortex**, is responsible for **executive control functions**, meaning nonautomatic actions that depend on decision making, planning, and attention. People whose prefrontal cortex has been damaged by physical trauma or stroke are impaired in executive control functions, and they often show abnormal emotions and excessive impulsiveness. The same clinical signs are seen in schizophrenia.

The prefrontal cortex is one of the last areas to mature in the entire brain. The reduction of gray matter and the increase in white matter occur here very late in adolescence. At this time, too, the fiber tracts that connect the prefrontal cortex with distant regions of the brain grow strongly.[4] The late development of these pathways may underlie the improved control over behavior as people transition from being adolescents to being adults. In light of both the known functions of the prefrontal cortex and its unique late development, it is perhaps not surprising that several abnormalities of structure and function have been reported in the prefrontal cortices of people who have schizophrenia.

To summarize, Daniel Weinberger and others believe that the key events leading to schizophrenia occur either before birth or in the infant child.[5] They say that an environmental event interacts with early brain development to produce a structural defect. The defect causes little or no problem in childhood, but when the brain is fine-tuned and updated during adolescence, the disruptive effects of the developmental glitch become apparent.

A minority view among scientists finds the evidence of an early developmental defect less than convincing. According to this alternative hypothesis, there is no brain abnormality until late adolescence or early adulthood. All that one needs to imagine, these scientists say, is an error in the reconfiguration that occurs during the final stages of brain development. Yet another opinion maintains that there is indeed an early defect but that there are no additional complications thereafter. In this view, the effects of the early defect simply accumulate over time as the brain grows. Eventually, the problems (erroneous connections) become so numerous and so pervasive that they produce a noticeable effect on behavior, and this usually happens around the time of adolescence.

Despite widespread support for the general *idea* that neurodevelopmental errors lie at the heart of schizophrenia, *proof* of the hypothesis is another matter. I have already written of certain genes with known roles in brain development that are associated, albeit weakly, with the risk of schizophrenia. In chapter 12, I will describe numerous brain anomalies that are associated with schizophrenia (including those in the prefrontal cortex), all of which *could* arise during neural development. The problem is, unless one can show that a brain anomaly appears *before* any symptoms of schizophrenia appear, there is no way of knowing whether the anomalies in the brains of people with schizophrenia are the *causes* of the behavioral symptoms or the *by-products* of the disease and its medications. Only one anomaly has passed this test, and that is the exaggerated reduction of gray matter during adolescence.

The finding has been replicated several times by different groups of investigators. A particularly convincing example comes from a recent study done in Scotland in which young people at high risk for schizophrenia were recruited together with another group of healthy control subjects.[6] None of the subjects had any symptoms of schizophrenia at the time of recruitment. The brains of all subjects were scanned every two years for a total of five times, as the subjects themselves were monitored for clinical signs of schizophrenia. All subjects lost cortical mass (largely gray matter) over the course of the study, but the high-risk subjects lost significantly more than did the healthy control subjects, particularly in the prefrontal lobe and the **temporal lobe**. Seventeen of the high-risk individuals developed schizophrenia, and the scans of these persons showed a greater loss of volume in the prefrontal cortex than did either the high-risk individuals who did not get schizophrenia or the healthy control subjects. Furthermore, in those subjects who became ill, the accelerated reduction of cortical volume began two to four years before the onset of the disease, and its progression correlated with the increased severity of symptoms. Because the high-risk subjects lost cortical volume before any became sick, the results suggest an early problem in neural development. Also, because the loss of volume continued at an even greater rate in those high-risk individuals who became sick, we can imagine that an additional error occurred near the onset of the disease. In other words, this study lends support to Weinberger's two-step version of the neurodevelopmental hypothesis.

The research described above illustrates some of the obstacles to proving any aspect of any version of the neurodevelopmental hypothesis. First of all, because researchers must use noninvasive methods, principally MRI imaging, it is impossible to look at numbers of neurons, numbers of synapses, numbers of **neurotransmitter receptors**, and levels of key neurochemicals. The resolution of even the best MRI scanners is no better than a couple of millimeters, which means that none of these features can be measured. Moreover, in prospective studies that continue for several years (10 years in the study described above), investigators have to deal with older scanning machines being replaced by newer models, and other technical changes, which together complicate comparisons between scans of single individuals at successive times.

There is also a problem in getting enough of the right kinds of human subjects. This is important because of the requirement for statistical power. For a prospective study in which it is unknown who is going to get schizophrenia, one would ordinarily need to recruit 1,000 people in order to study, on average, seven who later develop schizophrenia. Clearly, given the time and expense involved, this is impractical. The authors of one study described above overcame this problem by searching throughout Scotland for young, mentally healthy people who had two or more close relatives with schizophrenia. They had wanted to recruit 200 high-risk subjects but wound up with only 146. Even so, recruiting just the first 100 subjects "was a very labour-intensive process necessitating viewing of over 2,500 sets of case notes and approximately 500 home visits to patients and their families."[7] Lastly, performing experiments on the developing human brain is clearly out of bounds. Researchers cannot create brain abnormalities in order to test which specific disruptions cause which types of behavioral impairments.

Many of the foregoing obstacles can be overcome by using animals. With animals, but not humans, investigators can manipulate neurodevelopment to observe the consequences. Some interventions produce animals that act, in some ways, like humans with schizophrenia. Nobody claims that animals have hallucinations or delusions, and certainly not incoherent speech. However, the experiments can produce animals that are hyperactive, impulsive, socially inept, saddled with memory deficits, and prone to exaggerated responses to stress. The animals (typically rats or mice) demonstrating one or more of these traits are said to "model" human schizophrenia. The big advantage of animal models is that they allow investigators to test hypotheses about causes and effects. By manipulating selected genes, investigators can learn what roles these genes play in normal nervous system development and the disruptions that mutations in the genes may cause. By inducing certain of the brain abnormalities seen in the brains of people with schizophrenia, they can test which aberrant behaviors, if any, are caused by those abnormalities.

Other studies examine environmental causes and effects by subjecting pregnant animals to high levels of stress or exposing fetuses to viruses. In the majority of these experiments, it matters little that the rodent brain is not identical to the human brain or that the behaviors do not precisely match those of schizophrenia, as long as the experiments are able to prove a hypothesis true or false. Several experiments using animal models are discussed in chapter 12.

It is even possible to study schizophrenia using neither human subjects nor animals. Researchers are now able to study how genes and the environment affect neural development using laboratory cultures of neural networks grown in a Petri dish. A recent study illustrates the power of these techniques.[8] Fibroblasts, a type of cell found in connective tissue, were obtained from people with schizophrenia as well as from people who did not have schizophrenia. The fibroblasts, like all cells in the body, carry a complete set of a person's genes, both normal and variant. Incubating the fibroblasts in appropriate solutions transformed the cells into stem cells, and the stem cells were then induced to produce neurons. The young neurons formed small networks with seemingly normal anatomical and physiological properties.

A comparison of the neural networks made from people with schizophrenia and those derived from healthy human subjects revealed several significant differences. For example, the schizophrenia neurons had fewer branches, were less frequently connected to other neurons through synapses, and had reduced concentrations of several key synaptic proteins. Gene activity also differed in the two types of cultures. Nearly 600 genes had significantly different rates of activity (either more or less) in the schizophrenia neurons as compared with the normal neurons. Remarkably, when a commonly prescribed antipsychotic drug, clozapine (sold as Clozaril, Clopine, Lozapin, and other names), was added to the culture fluid, several aberrant features of the schizophrenia neurons were either eliminated or made nearly normal. In addition to their value for studying neural development, neurons grown in Petri dishes can be used to test antipsychotic drugs without the confounding influences of treatment histories, lifestyles, and individual reactions, and without experimenting on a single human or animal.

I need to end this chapter with a final note of caution regarding the neurodevelopmental hypothesis. At the beginning of the chapter I stated that the onset of schizophrenia peaks in the early twenties for men and in the late twenties for women. Thus, for both sexes, the peak ages for diagnosis roughly correspond to the final stages of brain development. However, a different picture emerges when we look at the total distribution of ages when schizophrenia begins, rather than at the peak ages. Approximately one-fifth of men and one-third of women are not diagnosed with schizophrenia until they are more than 30 years of age, by which time brain development is essentially complete in both sexes. This suggests that errors of neurodevelopment might not suffice as an explanation for schizophrenia, or at least that there are different causes in late-onset disease and early-onset disease. Moreover, there are differences between men and women.[9]

I have mentioned that women generally develop the disease a few years later than men. In addition, schizophrenia is about 30 percent less common in women than in men, and the symptoms are usually less severe in women. One clue that might hint at an explanation for these differences is the fact that women, but not men, show a secondary, late peak of onset, at ages 45 to 49 years. Because these ages correspond to the time of menopause or the approach of menopause, it has been suggested that the hormone estrogen protects women from schizophrenia so long as it is circulating at relatively high levels, perhaps by moderating the pruning of excess synapses. However, once estrogen concentrations fall, in menopause, women who have a predisposition for schizophrenia become vulnerable to the disease. This hypothesis could also explain the overall lower rate of schizophrenia and the generally milder symptoms in women compared to men.

SUMMARY

- Because the brain must be faithfully constructed according to a genetically defined program of development, and because schizophrenia typically becomes manifest near the end of a long period of brain maturation, schizophrenia is thought to be a disorder of nervous system development.

- Most experts believe that schizophrenia starts with a critical disruption of brain development very early in life, perhaps even before birth. The delayed appearance of schizophrenia, typically in late adolescence, is attributed either to the cumulative effects of the early developmental error or to the addition of another developmental error in adolescence.

- A protective influence from the hormone estrogen may explain the finding that, on average, women develop schizophrenia a few years later than men. As well, the appearance of a secondary peak of onset in women at ages 45–49, which is not seen in men, could be explained by the decrease in estrogen concentrations that follows menopause.

- The cerebral cortex normally undergoes major changes during adolescence. The amount of gray matter (neuronal cell bodies and dendrites) decreases, while the amount of white matter (axons) increases, and billions of synapses disappear. The prefrontal cortex, which controls several cognitive functions that are impaired in schizophrenia, is one of the last areas to exhibit such changes.

- Although many data are consistent with the neurodevelopmental hypothesis, the hypothesis has not yet been proved. It remains possible, for example, that a virus or other biological agent could attack an otherwise normal brain.

- It is important to establish causes and effects for suspected mechanisms. Prospective studies with people at high risk for schizophrenia have confirmed not only that high-risk individuals have smaller cortical volumes than mentally healthy people but also that the loss of cortical volume accelerates before the onset of disease.
- Animal models are useful for testing specific hypotheses under controlled experimental conditions. Manipulations performed early in life can cause animals to develop behavioral abnormalities that resemble schizophrenia symptoms or create brain abnormalities that likewise mimic those seen in brains of people with schizophrenia; some manipulations have both outcomes.

9

Two State Hospitals

With bills mounting fast from Edgemont Hospital and no improvement in Jim's condition, Mom and Dad decided to move my brother to the Norwalk State Hospital in southeast Los Angeles. I had recently begun my undergraduate studies at Stanford University, near San Francisco, and when I returned home on spring break, the three of us visited Jim at the hospital. Constructed in 1915, this facility sits on a large property of 162 acres. In the beginning, agricultural fields and a dairy farm on the property supplied the hospital with all the food it needed. Although food is now procured from the usual sources, a few of the old farm-style buildings still stand. We saw none of this architectural past as we pulled into the parking lot; all we saw was a modern tower built of brick, glass, and aluminum.

Jim may have moved from Edgemont to a different hospital, but he was still receiving electroconvulsive shocks. After all, an authority had recently written that "convulsive therapy now holds the field as the most effective single remedy in the whole range of psychiatry in relation to the number of patients deriving benefit from the treatment. Its use should not be restricted to the mental hospital."[1]

We were anxious to see how Jim was faring. Twice previously, Dad had driven us in his 1954 Chevy down the Santa Monica Freeway until it intersected with the Golden State Freeway near the city center. From there, he switched to the Golden State and drove on to Norwalk. On both occasions, we arrived at the hospital only to be told that Jim would not see us. These fruitless trips had been disappointing to say the least, so this time we phoned beforehand to find out whether he would welcome us. The report was positive, and we headed down the freeways again. In the main building, we rode an elevator and stepped out into a room that held the nurses' station and a seating area. Surprisingly, considering that the room was used by families when visiting their loved ones, there was absolutely no privacy. Utilitarian chairs were loosely arranged to accommodate small groups of people, but the room lacked partitions of any type. The entire space was dull and colorless, except for the orange plastic seats on the aluminum-framed chairs.

"We've come to see James Chase," said Dad through a small hole in the glass wall that surrounded the nurses' station. "We phoned earlier this morning."

"I'll ring for him," replied the nurse. "Wait over there until he comes out." The nurse gestured toward the chairs and returned to her paperwork. Three other visitors huddled silently at the far end of the room. We fixed our attention on a door near the nurses' station and waited. It was all too obvious what lay behind the door, constructed of thick glass reinforced with steel rods and heavily secured with locks. We waited. From time to time a nurse appeared with a patient, but not Jim. We wondered whether he had changed his mind. Then, finally, after nearly an hour, Jim walked through the door. From the vacant expression on his face and the slow, awkward gait, it was immediately apparent that he was not his usual self.

Mom hugged Jim, as she always did, and Jim stiffened up, also as expected. He was listless, and he had to be led to the chair that we were saving for him.

"It's so nice to see you dear," said Mom.

"Uh."

"How are you feeling?"

"Uh."

"I know that you had another treatment. You must be tired."

"Uh uh," Jim confirmed.

I was curious, so I asked, "Do you remember anything about the treatment?"

"No."

Next, it was Dad's turn. He did not like talking about Jim's shock treatments, in part because the idea horrified him and in part because he did not want to acknowledge that Jim was so sick that he needed such an extreme measure. He preferred to talk about everyday events that might be of interest to Jim.

"Tomorrow is the big game between UCLA and USC. Let's hope the Bruins lick 'em good this time. I have a lot of money at stake on this game. I gave Ted four points on a 37 cent bet." Dad liked to joke around; his friend Ted was a willing partner in the buffoonery. "I guess we don't have to ask who you will be rooting for, do we Jim?"

"I . . . you can . . . my school . . . go to win." Jim was mumbling in a barely audible voice. The words tumbled out like stones in a fast moving creek, his mind way ahead of his mouth.

Mom tried to help. "Slow down, Jim. Relax."

"I don't want to play football. Did you say Bruins? Brewing bears." Then, after a pause, "I don't know what I am saying. Confused. Too many thoughts. Confused."

Mom again tried to comfort him, "That's okay, dear, we understand."

I decided to change the subject. "Jim," I asked, "What have you been reading lately?" This was a stupid question, but what did I know about schizophrenia and electroconvulsive shock? I was just looking for a way to get Jim to talk. Clearly, he had not been reading anything at all, so his perfectly natural response to my question was a slow movement of his head from side to side, as if to say, "Sorry, but you don't understand."

Everyone was now feeling uncomfortable, and the strain on Jim was palpable. It was a symptom of his illness that he could not or would not talk about his feelings. Negative emotions built up in him until they exploded. Right now, Jim was feeling not just uncomfortable, but also disoriented, humiliated, and angry.

Ignoring the delicacy of the situation, Dad pressed on, asking, "How do you like it here? Have you made any new friends?"

With these questions, Jim fell from his psychological precipice. He rose from his seat, walked over to the nurses' station, and demanded that he be returned to the ward. He waited at the reinforced glass door until an attendant arrived to open it. Then, without even a glance at us, Jim disappeared into a fluorescent corridor on the other side of the door.

Electroconvulsive shock therapy is notorious for causing mental confusion and the loss of memories. Fortunately these effects were only temporary in Jim's case. Within a few days of our visit, Jim was back to his old (schizophrenic) self. Altogether he must have had about a dozen electroconvulsive shock treatments. On the whole, they neither harmed him nor did him any good.

In the intervals between shock treatments, when Jim was relatively lucid, he got talk therapy at Norwalk, and plenty of it. In a letter he wrote me from the hospital, he described the therapeutic schedule,

> They have a new regime here, under which you hardly have time to take a breath. In the mornings you work and in the afternoon you attend a barrage of therapy sessions. There is group psychotherapy, there is therapy with Dr. Bradley, there is Human Relations Therapy. I am beginning to wish they had a therapy for recovery from therapy. However, it is possible that out of all this some benefit may emerge. Incidentally, at the therapy session with Dr. Bradley last Friday we were talking about cars as expressions of masculinity.

Unfortunately, neither shock treatments nor talk therapy was able to ward off my brother's developing psychosis, so after a few months at Norwalk State Hospital, Jim was moved to another public facility, Camarillo State Hospital. The decision was made by the hospital authorities, not by our family. I assumed that he was being moved because Norwalk was not in the business of housing long-term patients, whereas Camarillo was. We learned the true reason for his transfer later, but in the meantime I was devastated by the news. Bad enough that Camarillo was located some 50 miles from our home. Much worse, was the hospital's dark reputation.

For me, Camarillo State Hospital was, above all else, the hospital in which the great jazz saxophonist Charles "Charlie" (Bird) Parker had been a patient. Addicted to heroin and alcohol, Parker was arrested and committed to Camarillo in the summer of 1946 after he set fire to his Los Angeles hotel room and ran naked through the lobby. He was 26 years old, the same age as Jim when *he* went to Camarillo. Parker spent six months at Camarillo detoxifying, playing in the hospital band, and tending a lettuce patch. To commemorate his time there, he composed a jazz piece titled "Relaxin' at Camarillo." After his release, he stayed clean for a while but then returned to his drug habit even as he continued to perform brilliantly. He died in New York City at age 34. Parker's story bore all the hallmarks of a legend: a musical genius condemned to stagnation in an isolated insane asylum accompanied by destitute madmen. I had absorbed the story as a fan of Parker's music and a connoisseur of jazz culture. It was only natural that I would shudder at the thought of Jim being admitted to Camarillo State Hospital.

In reality, the physical hospital was rather attractive. It was situated in a bucolic valley and built in the "mission revival style." And, like the Norwalk hospital, it had its own dairy and agricultural fields. Its red clay rooftops, courtyards, tiled fountains, and distinctive bell tower were spoiled only by their dilapidated condition and poor reputation. Mom and Dad must have seen enough of the place after delivering Jim for admission, because neither of them ever returned there to visit him. But I did.

Having arranged in advance that I would meet Jim in the "day room" at a certain hour, I walked directly from the entrance into a large atrium with a low ceiling. Jim was not yet there. Although I could see the sky through the high, curtained windows, the room itself was dark and eerily quiet, even with many patients there. Some of the patients were seated; others wandered about. Many of them were engaged in repetitive movements, whether shuffling their feet as they ambulated, rocking, or nodding their heads. Hardly any patients were engaged in conversation, but I made out a background noise of people mumbling to themselves.

I stood around for several minutes, growing more and more uncomfortable, and then I spotted Jim walking through a distant door. After greetings (no hugs), he directed me to a door that led out into a passageway crowded with patients. No sooner had we stepped into the passageway than a thin, elderly woman approached me asking for a cigarette. Like nearly everyone else in the room, she wore well-worn, drab clothing. I ignored her as best as I could, and Jim and I entered a courtyard where we sat down on a bench perched against a wall, giving us a good view of the large congregation gathered in the courtyard. There was more chatting here than in the atrium, but most of the patients seemed absorbed in their thoughts. A man seated near us moaned continuously as he rocked back and forth. Another fellow carried on as though he were Jesus (a common delusion). Many of the patients were smoking, and several approached me for a cigarette or a light. It was a scene similar to those I would encounter many times in the future, at other hospitals and custodial institutions, but there was a difference here. Perhaps because of my naiveté, I felt threatened.

Jim seemed calm, whereas I was wary among the other patients. Oddly, I felt safe only because I trusted the man sitting next to me, my brother. But how could he, with all his sensitivity and intelligence, not be agitated?

Looking around the courtyard, I asked him, "Do you know any of these people?"

"No."

"Have you been reading anything?"

"No."

"I stopped here on my way up to school."

"Oh. Stanford is a good school. What are you studying?"

"Psychology. It's pretty boring."

"Maybe you will switch majors," Jim replied. "I started out in chemistry, but I later switched to English literature."

"Why did you do that?"

"I don't remember. You're a good student. You'll do well at Stanford."

"I hope so," I said. "It's going okay so far."

We talked in fits and starts for about fifteen minutes, and then an attendant told us that we were all to leave the courtyard. I said goodbye to Jim in the atrium, exited to the parking lot, and drove north to Stanford University with tears in my eyes.

As events unfolded, my opinion of Camarillo State Hospital had to be drastically revised. Following my visit, Jim's condition gradually improved to the point where, six months later, he was living in an apartment in the nearby town of Ventura. Several years afterward, I learned the reason for the dramatic turnaround at Camarillo State Hospital. Far from being the backwater repository for the hopelessly insane that I imagined it to be, the hospital was in fact engaged in cutting-edge research on the treatment of schizophrenia. A new drug, chlorpromazine, had recently become available, and questions were being raised as to how it stacked up against current methods of treatment. To address this issue, the psychiatrists at the hospital initiated a study that operated under the plain title, the Schizophrenia Research Project.[2]

The carefully designed study set out to test which of five treatment options was most beneficial: **psychotherapy** (with a psychoanalytic orientation), drug therapy (using chlorpromazine), psychotherapy *plus* drugs, electroconvulsive shock, or social and environmental support. Jim might have been one of the patients included in the study, because it was conducted in the years 1959–1962, which includes the period of his stay. However, the study enrolled only 228 patients from a total of 6,900 people who were admitted to the hospital with a diagnosis of schizophrenia in those years (6,900!), so it is statistically unlikely that Jim was a participant. Nevertheless, I have no doubt that he benefited from the study's main finding, because he quickly got better.

The psychiatrists expressed themselves unequivocally in the summary of their study, "The results of our research demonstrate beyond reasonable doubt that drug therapy is the most effective single form of 'specific' treatment for the general run of schizophrenic hospital patient." And, "It is reasonably clear that electroconvulsive therapy cannot be considered to be desirable as an alternative or serious rival to drug therapy." As for psychotherapy, "at this stage of the illness, individual psychotherapy alone without drugs is an expensive and ineffective form of treatment that apparently adds little or nothing to conservative [nonmedical] therapies."[3] With these words, or rather with the implementation of the new program in the wards of Camarillo State Hospital, Jim was liberated from the frustrations of psychotherapy and the terrors of electroconvulsive shock. In their place, he received a medication that minimized the worst symptoms of his disease and provided him with many years of relative stability.

10

What Are the Treatment Options?

For every disease, there are dreams of finding a magic bullet, a treatment that completely cures the disease without causing any side effects. The idea was first floated early in the twentieth century by the German medical researcher Paul Ehrlich. He won the Nobel Prize in 1908 for his work in immunology, but he is also known for discovering the drug Salvarsan, which proved to be very effective in treating syphilis, a disease that was widespread and often fatal at the time. Salvarsan quickly became the treatment of choice for syphilis until it was superseded by penicillin.

The manner in which Ehrlich discovered Salvarsan is instructive because it shows why there is no magic bullet for schizophrenia, and why none is likely to be found. Ehrlich, like other researchers, knew that syphilis is caused by the bacterium *Treponema pallidum*. Unlike the others, however, Ehrlich realized that he could cure the disease if he could find a chemical that would selectively attach to the bacterium and kill it. So, he systematically tested a succession of compounds until, finally, with the 606th compound, he had a winner in Salvarsan. Because there is no single cause of schizophrenia, whether in the genome, in the environment, or even in the brain,[1] it is unlikely that any single drug could be completely effective against the disease, and in practice most people with schizophrenia receive more than a single drug. But drugs are not the only option. There are, in addition, physical therapies and psychosocial therapies.

Physical therapies have a long history in psychiatric medicine. In the Middle Ages, doctors imagined that they could remove a "stone of madness" to cure mental illnesses. In the eighteenth and nineteenth centuries, water baths, mustard plasters, fever cures, prolonged sleep, and physical punishments were all tried. Nothing suggests that any of these treatments worked. As late as the early 1930s, patients receiving a diagnosis of schizophrenia faced what amounted to "a death sentence, for the patient would be consigned to a life either cloistered at home, there to be locked in a bedroom and harangued by a distraught parent, or placed in an institution the joylessness of which it is difficult today to even imagine."[2] Shortly thereafter, a wave of new physical therapies emerged, two of which became notorious.

Lobotomies were surgical procedures that either removed a patient's frontal lobe or undercut that lobe's connections to the rest of the brain. Performed for the first time in Portugal in 1935, the operation had become widespread in the United States by the late 1940s. Most of the patients who received the lobotomies were highly agitated and difficult to manage before surgery, and the procedure was successful insofar as it had a tranquilizing effect. However, the operation deprived patients of a part of the brain that is responsible for some of humans' most highly evolved attributes. Following surgery, the lobotomized patients became lethargic, showed poor judgment, and often acted as though they had no social inhibitions. By the early 1950s, doctors came to understand that a lobotomy is, in fact, a savage and unethical assault on the human brain, and they stopped doing them. Just before the dangers were widely recognized, Dr. Egas Moniz was ironically awarded the Nobel Prize, in 1949, "for his discovery of the therapeutic value of leucotomy [lobotomy] in certain psychoses."

Electroconvulsive therapy, or ECT, does work, at least for some patients. The idea for therapeutic lobotomies originated in experiments on animals, but the precursors of electrical shock treatments for schizophrenia were trials involving other forms of physical therapy. In their fascinating telling of the story of ECT, the historians Edward Shorter and David Healy describe how, in 1933, a Viennese doctor named Manfred Sakel began experimenting with insulin injections as a cure for schizophrenia. Insulin, delivered in high doses, removes glucose from the blood and induces a coma. In the initial trials, the patients awoke from the coma feeling much better and exhibiting few symptoms of psychotic illness. The results were so good that insulin comas became something of a medical sensation. Dr. Sakel noticed, however, that in addition to the coma, his patients also developed epileptic-like convulsions. Consequently, a controversy ensued as to whether the beneficial effects of insulin therapy were due to the coma or the convulsions.

A Hungarian psychiatrist, Ladislaus Meduna, believed the convulsions were responsible, because his clinical observations suggested that patients with epilepsy never had schizophrenia and, conversely, that patients with schizophrenia never had epilepsy.[3] Seeking to induce seizures without inducing a coma, he decided to use a drug (camphor) that excites the brain. His first patient was a 33-year-old man who heard voices in his stomach and had spent the entire preceding year under bedcovers. On the morning after the last injection of camphor, the patient entered into a spirited conversation with the doctors and was surprised to learn that he had been in the hospital for four years. According to Dr. Meduna's own account of the aftermath, the patient felt so good that he escaped from the hospital, went home "and found out that the cousin living with his wife was not a relation at all but his wife's lover. He beat up the cousin and kicked him out of the house; proceeded to beat up his wife and told her that he . . . preferred to live in the state mental hospital where there is peace and honesty."[4] Later, in Rome, another doctor began using electrical currents instead of camphor to induce seizures, and ECT was born.

ECT was initially hailed as the "penicillin of psychiatry." One hospital found that 68 percent of 275 schizophrenia patients either recovered completely or were much improved after ECT. These results, however, signaled only a qualified success, because they applied only to patients who had been ill for six months or less. By contrast, the success rate was a mere 8 percent for patients who had been ill for two years or more. Also, the criteria for diagnosing schizophrenia in the mid-twentieth century were different from what they are today. In particular, catatonia, a motor condition characterized by either rigidity or constant agitation, was then considered a symptom of schizophrenia, but it is now associated with several different psychiatric disorders. Thus, by current definitions, many of the cases designated as "schizophrenia" in the early ECT trials were not really schizophrenia. All things considered, contemporary psychiatrists find ECT of limited value in treating schizo-phrenia, though it can be effective when used in conjunction with drug therapies, especially in first-episode cases and with patients who are otherwise unresponsive to drugs. ECT is more frequently used in the treatment of depression, bipolar disease, and catatonia.

Many people associate ECT with lobotomy and consider both of them as inhuman treatments. They think that ECT is dangerous and causes bad side effects. However, the truth of the matter is that whereas lobotomy deserves its repugnant reputation, ECT does not. The public perception of ECT constitutes a prime example of medical misinformation. Earlier concerns over such problems as fractured bones (from uncontrolled movements during seizures), anxiety, lack of informed consent, and indiscriminate administration are no longer valid, and techniques have gotten better and better. The only major side effect is a temporary memory deficit that mainly affects memories of recent events. The claim that ECT causes "brain damage" is totally unfounded. Unfortunately, the public's image of ECT is too often based on the film *One Flew over the Cuckoo's Nest*, where the portrayal of ECT bears little resemblance to the modern procedure. Summing up their views on the controversial nature of ECT, the authors Shorter and Healy remark, "It is hard in fact to think of anywhere where the mismatch between rhetoric and reality is as great as it has been in the history of ECT."[5]

Today, new types of physical therapies for mental illnesses are being tested. Transcranial magnetic stimulation (TMS) generates small electrical currents within confined regions of the brain using external magnets; the currents excite some local neurons while inhibiting others. Another procedure, known as deep brain stimulation, requires that fine wire electrodes be implanted in the brain. As with TMS, the goal is to either stimulate or inhibit neurons. By inserting electrodes rather than using external magnetic devices, the action can be localized with greater precision. Also, because less equipment is needed, the method can be used with ambulatory patients. However, no one wants to walk around with wires coming out their heads. And besides, although TMS and deep brain stimulation both look promising as treatments for depression, neither seems to be effective in schizophrenia.

With physical therapies sidelined, at least so far as schizophrenia is concerned, current treatment programs rely heavily on pharmaceutical products. The first drug shown to be truly effective against schizophrenia was chlorpromazine. It was developed in France in 1950 as an antihistamine.[6] Antihistamines are seen today as over-the-counter remedies for allergies, but they were once considered useful in the management of many conditions, including those relating to cardiovascular, gynecological, obstetrical, and neurological complaints. Fittingly, the original trade name for chlorpromazine was Largactil, meaning "with a large or broad action."

The discoverer of chlorpromazine, Dr. Henri Laborit, was a surgeon in the French navy. In early trials, Laborit observed that the drug made surgical patients indifferent to their surroundings and to their own bodies. Hence, he began to use it as a sedative agent in surgeries and sleep therapies; it was administered as part of an anesthetic "cocktail." The discovery of its benefits for psychiatric patients happened in 1952, and quite by accident. It was customary, at the Hôpital Sainte-Anne in Paris, to literally cool down the most highly agitated patients by putting them in ice baths. The patients were given chlorpromazine before being placed in the baths. When it developed that the demand for ice exceeded the capacity of the pharmacy to supply it, the nurses simply gave chlorpromazine without any ice bath, *et voilà*, the calming effect was no different than if the ice bath had been included. Once the psychiatrists confirmed the benefits of chlorpromazine, they too began to use it "without theorizing about what it might be doing or why. The effects of the new treatment were extraordinary."[7]

Several years passed before physicians started using chlorpromazine in North American hospitals. It was successfully tested in Toronto and Montreal as early as 1953, but it was not sold in North America until 1955, at which time it was licensed as an antiemetic (antivomiting drug) and marketed as Thorazine. As soon as clinical trials in the United States confirmed the Canadian results, Thorazine became the drug of choice for treating schizophrenia throughout the continent.

Despite its commercial success, however, chlorpromazine is only a partial remedy for schizophrenia, because it leaves many symptoms unaffected. Chlorpromazine works well in suppressing the positive symptoms—hence its apparent calming effect—but it does little to improve the negative symptoms. Also, chlorpromazine can produce some nasty side effects. Patients who have been on chlorpromazine for long periods can develop stiffened bodies and engage in repetitive motor actions. Several other drugs that are closely related to chlorpromazine, like haloperidol (Haldol), have similar effects and similar limitations.

Thus, while chlorpromazine and its kin were big commercial successes, they fell short of what patients needed. Acknowledging this reality, the pharmaceutical industry tried to find new antipsychotic drugs. From laboratory investigations, they suspected that chlorpromazine worked by affecting the neurotransmitter dopamine. Eventually, a consensus grew among scientists that chlorpromazine blocks one of the two main receptors for dopamine and that, in doing so, it corrects an excess of dopamine that lies at the heart of schizophrenia's positive symptoms. Meanwhile, other research suggested that the neurotransmitter serotonin is implicated in the negative symptoms. With these insights in hand, the pharmacologists set out to design a new drug that would target not only dopamine but also serotonin. The result was a new class of "atypical" or "second generation" antipsychotic drugs, of which clozapine (Clozaril) is the best known.

Despite their heavy promotion by drug companies, the second generation of antipsychotic drugs has turned out to be only slightly better than the first generation. On average, they are about equally effective in reducing positive symptoms, but they have the advantage of causing fewer motor system side effects. None provides significant relief from schizophrenia's negative symptoms. Clozapine often works to control positive symptoms when no other drug is effective, but it carries the significant risk of lowering white blood cell counts; this is a potentially lethal condition that must be carefully guarded against through scheduled blood monitoring. Other side effects are common with second-generation drugs but differ from drug to drug. Weight gain, sedation, and high blood sugar levels are side effects of many of the drugs, while excessive salivation is unique to clozapine. Following on the disappointment of the atypical drugs, the search continues for an ideal antipsychotic medication. In total, more than 60 drugs are currently available.[8] Psychiatrists know that none of these drugs is "best" for schizophrenia, and they generally choose the most appropriate drug, or drugs, for each patient depending on his or her symptoms and clinical history.

Every pharmaceutical company dreams of developing a drug that eliminates the negative symptoms of schizophrenia, to gain credit for the achievement and to ensure a steady revenue stream. With this goal in mind, the pharmaceutical firms are designing new molecules. In one or another clinical trial, they have targeted all of the brain's neurotransmitters—namely, dopamine, acetylcholine, glutamate, serotonin, gamma aminobutyric acid (GABA), histamine, and glycine, as well as several **neuropeptides**.

In contrast to earlier drugs that act on the targeted neurotransmitter wherever it is present in the brain, the newer drugs can have more local actions. They do so by interfering with the process in which the neurotransmitter molecules are bound by, or captured by, receptor molecules embedded in the membranes of the receiving cells. Each neurotransmitter is bound by a family of related, but molecularly distinct, receptor molecules. For example, there are at least 17 different receptor types for serotonin, many of which can be selectively targeted by drugs.[9] Because different receptor types are present in different regions of the brain, it is possible to block, say, serotonin in one region while leaving its functions unaffected in all other regions of the brain. And yet, despite the power and elegance of the approach, none of the new drugs is dramatically more effective than even the first-generation antipsychotics in relieving negative symptoms.

Unfortunately, the psychological, cognitive, and behavioral functions that are disturbed in schizophrenia are served by some of the most highly evolved parts of the human brain. The neural circuits are complex on both grand and minute scales, and the physiological responses are supported by a vast array of chemical interactions. When one adds to this scenario the fact that the brains of people with schizophrenia contain numerous chemical abnormalities, it seems unlikely, on present evidence, that any crude pharmacological alteration of the brain's chemistry could eliminate all the symptoms of schizophrenia. The pharmacological approach—no matter how finely tuned—may be too blunt and come too late to correct the underlying neurodevelopmental defects.

The psychological and social methods aim primarily at supporting patients rather than treating the disease. Some advocates, however, go further. For example, the anthropologist Tanya Marie Luhrmann writes, "Clients are encouraged to take their medication, of course, but the real therapeutic change is thought to come through something social: something people learn to do, say, and believe."[10] The psychosocial methods are most effective in alleviating negative symptoms and boosting cognitive functions. There is a variety of approaches. The cognitive-behavioral approach encourages patients to adopt a reasoned attitude in respect to the illness. Although a few reports have claimed that cognitive-behavioral therapy reduces the frequency of hallucinations and delusions, other reports are contradictory; on the whole, the benefits appear to be "modest at best."[11] A technique called loving-kindness meditation is based on Buddhist principles; it shows promise for decreasing negative symptoms, while increasing the frequency and intensity of positive emotions. Brain-training video games represent a very different approach. Designed by a distinguished neuroscientist, these innovative tools are now sold as a commercial package. The company marketing the product claims that it boosts cognitive functions in such areas as problem solving, short-term memory, and recognition of social signals.[12]

Other therapies seek to educate patients about their illnesses or teach explicit social and practical skills that can benefit the patients in their everyday lives. In general, the psychosocial therapies that involve the patient's family are the most effective. For example, a group of Spanish patients received family-based psychosocial therapy while also taking antipsychotic drugs. After two years of treatment, the progress of these patients was compared with that of a control group in which patients received antipsychotic drugs but no family-based psychosocial therapy. After analyzing the results, the investigators concluded, "Family intervention significantly reduced the number of clinical relapses, major incidents, positive and negative symptoms and admissions to hospital, improved social functioning and relieved family burden, as compared with standard treatment."[13]

Can we expect to see significantly better therapies in the future? The answer for the near term, unfortunately, is no, but in the long term, yes. Unlike some other diseases, schizophrenia is not caused by a single genetic mutation, a single biochemical problem, or a single anatomical anomaly. It manifests itself in a variety of brain pathologies that are distributed in several regions of the brain and that affect both tiny synaptic connections and large network structures. Thus, it is very difficult to attack. Of the three types of therapy—physical, pharmacological, and psychosocial—only the pharmacological therapies offer any real hope for major breakthroughs, and only then if pharmacology teams up with genetics. In the epilogue, I will highlight some of the potential benefits of combining genetic and pharmacological approaches.

SUMMARY

- Electroconvulsive therapy has an undeserved negative reputation. Although it has ceased to be a mainstream therapy, ECT remains useful in the early stages of schizophrenia, in the treatment of drug-resistant cases, and when symptoms include catatonia.
- Transcranial magnetic stimulation and deep brain stimulation are not effective for treating schizophrenia, although they might benefit people with depression.
- Drugs are the most powerful instruments in the therapeutic tool box. When chlorpromazine (Thorazine) was accidently discovered to calm otherwise unmanageable patients, it quickly transformed the treatment of schizophrenia and ushered in the first generation of antipsychotic drugs. All medications of this type work by targeting dopamine neurotransmission.
- The second-generation drugs target multiple neurotransmitters, usually dopamine plus serotonin. As well, many of these medications act selectively on subtypes of neurotransmitter receptors, thus enabling more specific effects. While the newer drugs tend to have less severe side effects, they are not significantly more effective in reducing symptoms and improving function than the older, first-generation drugs.
- In general, current drugs suppress the positive symptoms of schizophrenia (paranoia, delusions, hallucinations) but have little or no effect on the negative symptoms (reduced affect, diminished social

life, poverty of thought) or on cognitive impairments (memory, attention, planning).

- Psychological and social therapies are mainly used in conjunction with drugs, where they can alleviate negative symptoms and boost cognitive functions. Patients often benefit from explicit instruction in compensatory behaviors and practical skills. Family-based interventions are especially effective.

11

A Conversation in a Park

Within months of first receiving his antipsychotic medications, Jim was out of Camarillo State Hospital and living in what is referred to as a halfway house, where he was about one-half independent and one-half assisted by social workers associated with the hospital. Everyone in the family was relieved to have Jim out of the hospital, and once his supervisors saw that he was holding things together well enough, they approved a move closer to home. Thus began a hopeful period in which Jim experimented with independent living. My parents set him up in an apartment in Santa Monica, and he was given a part-time job in the library of the Neuropsychiatric Institute and Hospital at UCLA, thanks to the folks in the clinic where he was an outpatient. Although he was managing his own affairs, more or less, he was emotionally unstable, poorly motivated, and prone to embarrassing public displays. Time and time again, some little annoyance would lead to a bigger problem, and before long he would be in real trouble.

On one occasion, I was called upon to retrieve Jim from a Bob's Big Boy restaurant near his apartment. He had been involved in a dustup with another customer. I apologized to the manager and drove Jim back to his apartment. Scenes such as this caused Jim, inevitably, it seems, to lose his job at the library. As well, they made it impossible for him to continue living in his current accommodations. Over the following several years, he moved through four more apartments in Santa Monica and one in Hollywood. Each time, after being removed from a residence after a psychiatric crisis, he would go to the UCLA Neuropsychiatric Hospital for a period of "cooling off." Once Jim stabilized, Dad would help him move into another apartment, where the cycle would begin again. On the whole, Jim was less psychotic now than before his stay at Camarillo (hence, before chlorpromazine), and he was more upbeat in mood, so we had hope that he might completely recover. But, with the repeated setbacks, our hopes faded. We gradually came to accept that Jim could not live by himself. For the remainder of his life, my brother would live in psychiatric board-and-care residences interspersed with brief stays in psychiatric hospitals when necessary.

Once, during the hopeful period mentioned above, Mom, Dad, and I spent the day in an idyllic oasis named Will Rogers State Historic Park. Will Rogers was a wildly popular actor and media personality in the early 1930s, and Mom and Dad were big fans. Situated on nearly 200 acres of hilly terrain overlooking the Pacific Ocean, the park was formerly the site of Will Rogers's home and private ranch. It is a lovely, quiet place with cultivated gardens and wild habitat, walking trails, and the scent of the giant eucalyptus trees surrounding the green polo field. In earlier years, when Jim was still okay, Mom would pack a lunch in her wicker basket, and we would enjoy a meal before hiking the trails or just relaxing on the grass. The mood on this particular occasion, however, was decidedly more somber. After lunch, Mom and I struck up a conversation.

"Mom," I said, "What do you think is the problem with Jim?"

"Well, we've got to accept that Jim has a mental illness."

"I know that, Mom, but does it mean that there is something wrong with his mind? I think Jim is thoughtful and very smart. After all, he's a graduate student at UCLA, isn't he?"

"Of course he is, Ron dear. Jim's intellect is perfectly fine—there's nothing wrong with *that*. What is wrong is some of his ideas, and how they tie up with his emotions. Some of his ideas are clearly not realistic. You know too that he gets depressed and angry. The doctors say that certain events in his childhood—they won't say which ones—made him nervous, and because he couldn't resolve these issues, his mind got messed up. It might even have had something to do with our family situation, how Dad and I treated Jim . . . I don't know. If you're interested in these things, you might like to read a new book called *The Vital Balance*. The author is one of America's most distinguished psychiatrists,

Dr. Karl Menninger. He and his brother run a large clinic in Topeka, Kansas. According to Dr. Menninger, nearly everyone has some degree of mental illness. It is just the result of how we are brought up. We all try to cope with life's stresses by creating a balance in the mind. Unfortunately, some of us do not achieve a very good balance, and that is what we call mental illness. Depending on how inadequate the balance is, the mental illness may be minor or serious. I'm afraid in Jim's case, it is rather severe."

"I don't understand what he means by 'balance.' Is it what Dad is always talking about, the 'golden mean' and 'everything in moderation,' which Dad says comes from Socrates?"

"Sort of, Ron, but it's more than that. You can think of it as involving conflicts. Sometimes a mother tells the child to act in a certain way, and then later, maybe in a different way, the mother tells the child the opposite. Or, the mother might say one thing and the father says the opposite. In that situation, the father might even punish the child for something that the mother had earlier told him to do. There is a smart fellow up near San Francisco by the name of Gregory Bateson who calls these types of conflicts 'double binds.' According to him, if a child has to constantly figure out what to do in the face of conflicting demands, he'll grow up with confused thinking, which can lead to schizophrenia. Who knows, such a thing could have happened with Jim, but frankly, I think Bateson misses the point about conflicts. I think they lie deeper than what he says.

"I go along with Sigmund Freud, who says that most conflicts are unconscious—we are not really aware of them. Our basic instincts, like sex and aggression, are in the unconscious. The instincts are very strong, but a person can have equally strong moral standards, so conflicts can arise between our drives and our morals. In the ancient Greek legend, a boy named Oedipus loved his mother and was jealous of his father. Freud thinks that even modern-day kids have these feelings. He thinks that boys unconsciously want to have sex with their mothers, which, obviously, they cannot do. So, with a conflict like that, a boy has trouble, that's for sure."

"Mom," I said, "you're not really suggesting that Jim has an Oedipus conflict, are you?"

"No. But, really, who am I to say? Remember, Freud tells us that we bury our conflicts deep in our unconscious minds. Sometimes this works out okay, but in other cases, the repressed conflicts fester and cause problems. So, yes, Jim could very well have an Oedipus conflict and, for that matter, so could you."

"Oh, come on . . . that's ridiculous!"

I tried to peer into my unconscious mind to find out if I did want to have sex with my mother. I was at first relieved to discover a strong negative reaction, but then I realized that Freud would have predicted no less. After all, repression works to hide such urges from our awareness. To bring them up from the emotional underworld into the light of consciousness requires the heavy work of psychoanalysis. But I was confused. Although I had a pretty good idea of what consciousness is, I couldn't get a grip on unconsciousness. Is it part of the mind, like consciousness, or is it something different, maybe unmind? And, for that matter, what *is* the mind?

As Mom told me that day in Will Rogers Park, Freud divides the mind into three parts. First there is the ego, which roughly corresponds to our conscious self. It is the rational part that directs our day-to-day activities. Then there is the id. Both the id and the third part, the superego, are unconscious. Basic human drives, like hunger, aggression, and sex are all in the id. Freud believed that sex is just part of a larger life force, which he called the libido. Now we come to the superego. It contains moral standards. We can think of it as our conscience. Because the superego is constantly trying to reign in the ego and the id, both of which have their own agendas, tensions arise and unconscious conflicts develop. Psychoanalysis helps us to get insights into the workings of our ids, egos, and superegos. When psychoanalysis works—and it does require a lot of work—we can each discover our own particular conflicts and resolve them.

Okay, I thought, so Freud believes the mind has three parts. But is the mind in the brain, or is it separate from the brain? Is it a *thing* like the brain is a *thing*?

Mom replied that the mind is what makes us aware of things. It is consciousness, the awareness of the world around us, and self-consciousness, the awareness of ourselves. The mind, she said, is responsible for all our experiences in the park. "Just think about the *greenness* of the grass and the *blueness* of the sky. Those special feelings aroused by the colors must be in the mind because the only things in the brain are neurons and fluids. There is a certain summer odor here as well, thanks to the grass cuttings and all the beautiful flowers. The feeling of that odor is also in the mind. And, to answer your question, yes, the mind is in the brain."

Mom was getting annoyed with my naive questions, but I pressed her on this point anyway. "What do you mean, the mind is *in* the brain? You said that there are only neurons in the brain, and blood vessels, and stuff like that? If the mind is not made of those things, what *is* it made of?"

"I don't know what the mind is made of," she answered, "what is important is that the mind and the brain work together, like your lungs and your muscles when you're running your races. Most of the time, except when you're sleeping or otherwise unconscious, the mind controls the brain. You feel something, you think about it, and then you decide what to do. All of that happens in your mind. Once the mind decides on a course of action, it instructs the brain to cause contractions in the appropriate muscles."

To drive home her argument, she challenged me with a practical demonstration. "Ron, if you don't believe what I am saying, let's try a little experiment. It's very simple. I just want you to lift one of your arms above your head. Take your time to decide which arm you want to lift, and when I say 'go,' do it."

I waited for her signal, and then raised my left arm.

"Well, you see," she said. "It's about free will. Your mind decided to move your arm—your left arm—and you did it. Your arm lay still until your mind issued the command. It's pretty obvious, isn't it?"

I had to admit that this evidence was compelling, but there were still things I didn't understand. Since you can't touch the mind or see it, it can't be a solid thing like the brain. So, is it like air? Or is it a bunch of little electrons flying around in the brain? How can the mind possibly control what the brain does if it isn't a physical thing like the brain? All those neurons . . . how does the mind get the right ones to fire their electrical sparks at exactly the right time?

Mom had clearly had enough of this conversation. She wanted to put an end to it, to stroll quietly in the gardens of the park, so she attempted

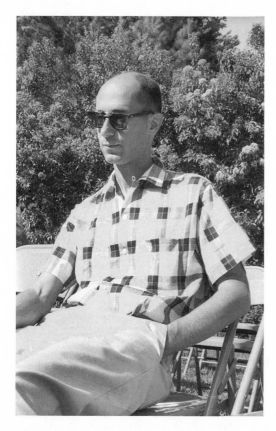

Jim, 1964

a summing up. "A little while ago you asked me what is wrong with Jim. I can only repeat what I said before. For whatever reason, there is some conflict or some wrong way of thinking that makes it difficult for him to behave like normal people. I know you suspect that there is something wrong with his brain, but I can tell you, I've spoken to several doctors about this. They've read the studies that looked for abnormal anatomies, altered chemistries, and electrical malfunctions in the brains of mentally ill persons. They could not tell me of a single physical correlate of Jim's behavioral and psychological symptoms. If these clever researchers can't see anything in their fancy microscopes, Jim's problem must lie in his mind, not in his brain. He has an illness of the mind."

Mom reached out and took my hand. "Come on, Ron, let's go for a walk."

12

Is Mental Illness in the Mind or in the Brain?

For there to be an illness of the mind, there must first be a mind, a thing different and separate from the brain. Otherwise, we should instead speak of brain illnesses. Intuition leads us to believe that we do have a mind, but it was not until the seventeenth-century philosopher René Descartes constructed an influential argument for the mind's independence from the brain that people began to take the idea seriously. With passionate assertions, Descartes gave an authoritative voice to the ancient philosophy of **dualism**, the belief that humans consist of both body and mind:

> I noticed that, while I was trying to think that everything was false, it was necessary that I, who was thinking this, should be something. And observing that this truth: *I think, therefore I am*, was so firm and secure that all the most extravagant suppositions of the skeptics were not capable of overthrowing it, I judged that I should not scruple to accept it as the first principle of the philosophy that I was seeking.

And:

> I knew that I was a substance whose whole essence or nature is only that of thinking, and which, in order to exist, has no need of any place, nor depends on any material thing. Thus this "I," that is to say the soul by which I am what I am, is entirely distinct from the body.[1]

About two hundred years later, the term *mental illness* appeared for the first time in Emily Brontë's novel *Wuthering Heights*. Although she intended it only as a metaphor, the term was interpreted literally by both physicians and the public, and that which had previously been known as madness became an illness *of the mind*.

Despite dualism's intuitive appeal, it is almost surely incorrect as a philosophy of mind. Beginning in the nineteenth century and continuing to the present, serious philosophers have overwhelmingly rejected the idea. They point out that it is plainly illogical to go from saying that one cannot think without existing to the claim that one's whole essence is to think. Just because Descartes says he is certain about these things does not mean that they are true. And then there is the little matter of the mind governing the brain. If the mind and the brain were truly separate "things," how could the nonphysical states of mind like desires, intentions, and plans possibly cause physiological activity in the brain? No one has been able to come up with a plausible explanation for how this could happen, despite the attempts of some bright philosophers and neuroscientists. Finally, Descartes's claim that the mind "has no need of any place, nor depends on any material thing" is obviously false, unless one believes in ghosts, telepathy, and reincarnation.[2]

Most contemporary philosophers say that the world contains only physical things and that which we refer to as the mind is simply an aspect of, or the result of, the brain's physiological activity. Hence, mental illnesses are *brain illnesses*; the problem is in the brain, not in the mind. This is not a new claim. It was stated as early as the fifth century B.C. by Hippocrates, the so-called father of modern medicine:

> Men ought to know that from nothing else but the brain come joys, delights, laughter and sports, and sorrows, griefs, despondency, and lamentations. . . . And by the same organ we become mad and delirious, and fears and terrors assail us, some by night, and some by day, and dreams and untimely wanderings, and cares that are not suitable, and ignorance of present circumstances, desuetude, and unskillfulness. All these things we endure from the brain, when it is not healthy.[3]

Notwithstanding the long history of biological psychiatry that began with Hippocrates, there have always been physicians who insisted either that mental illnesses are indeed *in the mind* or, more radically, that they do not even exist. One psychiatrist, Thomas Szasz, has taken both positions. In his widely read book with the audacious title

The Myth of Mental Illness,[4] he insisted that "mental illnesses" are nothing but imaginary disorders conceived for the purpose of enforcing social norms of behavior. Later, writing specifically about schizophrenia, he softened his position, but only slightly. In 1976 he wrote, "There is at present no demonstrable histopathological or pathophysiological evidence to support the claim that schizophrenia is a disease. Indeed, if there were any, the supporters of this claim would be the first to assert that schizophrenia is not a mental disease but a brain disease."[5] As I write now, more than 35 years later, there is overwhelming evidence of pathology in the brains of people with schizophrenia, and few informed people deny that schizophrenia is indeed a brain disease.

Every year, thousands of articles about schizophrenia are published in the research literature, some truly meaningful and others reporting trivial or misleading results. Scientists take seriously only the results that are obtained using rigorous methods, that have large effects, and that are replicated in multiple independent studies. Bearing in mind these criteria, I will now summarize the most important evidence for the neurobiological basis of schizophrenia.

Neuroscientists operate on the assumption that a genetic disposition combines with an environmental influence to produce abnormalities in the brain, which then cause schizophrenia. Most researchers believe that the brain is damaged during its development, and all researchers are guided by the abnormalities that they, or others, find in the brains of adults who have schizophrenia. Such signs of abnormality, called **biomarkers**, can be found in both living brains, using noninvasive brain scans, and the brains of deceased persons, using postmortem examinations.

As I mentioned previously, imaging methods can distinguish gray matter (mainly cell bodies and dendrites) and white matter (mainly axons) in living brains. These studies consistently find that people with schizophrenia have less gray matter than people who do not have schizophrenia, especially in the prefrontal lobe and the temporal lobe. Thus, the cortex is slightly thinner in people who have schizophrenia. Another highly reliable finding is that the fluid-filled spaces in the brain, called ventricles, are enlarged in people with schizophrenia.

Putting these two results together, it seems likely that the ventricles expand to take up space vacated by the thinned cortex. It is not known why the cortex is thinner, or how this anatomical feature explains the symptoms of schizophrenia, but the findings are consistent with the idea that a neurodevelopmental defect lies at the root of schizophrenia. Importantly, both the reduced gray matter and the enlarged ventricles are evident soon after the initial diagnosis, and in some cases even before the patients receive any antipsychotic medications. This means that the observed changes are likely a consequence of the disease itself, and not the result of either medications or the lifestyles of people with schizophrenia. Moreover, these abnormal brain structures seem to have a genetic basis.[6]

The white matter of the brain is another source of biomarkers. It is composed of axons, those slender extensions of nerve cells that connect different regions of the cerebral cortex with one another and connect the cortex with other parts of the brain. Estimates put the total length of all the axons in the brain at around 150,000 kilometers. The axons tend to bundle together in large masses that appear white because of the axons' fatty coverings, made from a substance called myelin. In most cases, a single bundle will contain some axons headed in one direction and others headed in the opposite direction, so the bundles usually support two-way communications.

With magnetic resonance imaging, it is possible to measure the diffusion of water particles along the white matter pathways, which in turn gives a measure of their structural integrity. When the white matter in the brains of people with schizophrenia is examined in this manner, the water particles consistently move at a slower rate than in healthy subjects. This finding indicates some type of structural defect—perhaps in the axons themselves, perhaps in their myelin, or perhaps in the overall organization of the bundles. In any case, the abnormal appearance of the white matter is a prominent biomarker for schizophrenia.

Because one of the functions of the white matter is to coordinate the activities of distant brain parts, researchers have also looked at the *physiological* integrity of the pathways in brains of people with schizophrenia, and here again they found an intriguing biomarker. In normal brains, a white matter connection allows the electrical activities of the **hippocampus** and the prefrontal lobe to be tightly synchronized. In schizophrenia, however, the degree of synchrony is much less. This finding is especially significant because the prefrontal lobe is already in the schizophrenia spotlight for other reasons.

To see whether there is a genetic basis for the impairment of hippocampal-prefrontal synchrony, a group of geneticists engineered a mouse to carry one of the risk factors for schizophrenia, a partial deletion of human chromosome 22. The synchrony was "drastically reduced" in these mice. Furthermore, the experimental animals were significantly impaired when tested on a simple memory task.[7] Another study examined the synchrony between the hippocampus and the prefrontal cortex in an animal model of schizophrenia. In this model, young rats show "a syndrome of structural, functional, and behavioural schizophrenia-like abnormalities" when, before birthing, the pregnant mothers are injected with a substance that activates the immune system.[8] It turns out that the synchrony between the hippocampus and the prefrontal cortex is disrupted in these schizophrenic-like rats. All together, the studies discussed here suggest that abnormalities in white matter are highly relevant biomarkers for schizophrenia.

Other biomarkers are seen after death when the whole brain, or parts of the brain, are cut into thin slices and examined under a microscope. This type of research was energetically pursued in the nineteenth century and remains a staple of fundamental neuroscience today. Alois Alzheimer was using postmortem brain tissues to research psychiatric disorders when he discovered the degenerative disease of aging that now carries his name. For schizophrenia, a useful result from the postmortem studies has been to confirm the findings relating to thinned cortices and enlarged ventricles that were noted above. In addition, postmortem anatomical studies have found that one specific type of neuron (found in the white matter) is abnormally distributed, another type of neuron (in the hippocampus) is unusually small, and a third type (in the hippocampus and the prefrontal cortex) is reduced in numbers. Again, all these results point to a problem in the development of the brain.

Postmortem brains can also be used for chemical studies. An important application involves measuring the protein content of schizophrenia specimens compared to nonschizophrenia specimens. Rather than measuring the total amount of protein, which would be only mildly informative, the investigations gather data on individual "species" of protein.[9] The human body contains about 20,000 different proteins, and most of them are present in the brain. In one study that focused on the temporal lobe, 37 proteins were found at significantly different concentrations in the brains of people with schizophrenia versus in the brains of people who do not have schizophrenia. For some proteins, the concentrations in the diseased brains were much lower than in the healthy brains, while for other proteins the opposite was true. Another study analyzed 1,800 proteins in the prefrontal cortex; it found significantly different concentrations for 67 proteins.[10]

The proteins identified in these studies have a variety of functions. In the prefrontal cortex, proteins involved in the immune system were strongly represented, which lends support to the idea that infections have a role in initiating schizophrenia. Among the other proteins implicated by these studies are some that maintain the fatty myelin sheaths around axons; quite possibly, reductions in the amounts of these proteins could account for the abnormalities observed in white matter pathways.

The postmortem findings that have attracted the most interest are those that relate to neurotransmitters, and this is because many researchers believe that neurotransmitters are somehow central to understanding schizophrenia. Dopamine was the first neurotransmitter to draw attention, after it was discovered that chlorpromazine and all the other first-generation drugs block one of the two main types of dopamine receptor molecules. From this fact grew the hypothesis that schizophrenia is caused by an excess of dopamine neurotransmission. Support for the idea came from the observation that amphetamine, a psychological and physical stimulant, releases dopamine in the brain; amphetamine can also produce schizophrenia-like symptoms in people who have no disease.

However, postmortem data, together with other evidence, have greatly complicated the picture of neurotransmitter involvement in schizophrenia. For starters, the postmortem results for dopamine receptors are inconclusive, because different results are obtained depending on the method used, and all the data are affected by the medications taken by the patients before they die. Also, additional neurotransmitters have been implicated. While some evidence points to serotonin, acetylcholine, and still other transmitters, it is glutamate and gamma-aminobutyric acid (GABA) that have spurred the most research.[11] The focus on glutamate and GABA has led to a detailed hypothesis that explains at least some aspects of schizophrenia, as described below.

Several types of observations implicate glutamate, the principal excitatory neurotransmitter, in schizophrenia. For one, pharmacological **antagonists** of glutamate produce schizophrenia-like symptoms in normal volunteers.[12] The effective antagonists include phencyclidine (PCP), dizocilpine (MK801), and ketamine, all of which are medical anesthetics, but also street, or recreational, drugs. In contrast to amphetamine, which triggers only positive symptoms, the glutamate antagonists induce both positive symptoms (psychosis) and negative symptoms (social withdrawal and memory deficits). Glutamate is also implicated by postmortem studies that show that schizophrenia brains contain fewer glutamate receptors than do normal brains. And finally, when glutamate transmission is impaired by genetic manipulations in experimental mice, the animals develop schizophrenic-like symptoms.

GABA is the main inhibitory transmitter in the brain. The case for its involvement comes primarily from postmortem studies, which report substantially lower concentrations of the transmitter in the brains of people with schizophrenia compared to the brains of people who do not have schizophrenia. As well, the enzyme that is responsible for synthesizing GABA and a protein that is necessary for its release are also found at reduced levels in the brains of people with schizophrenia. Not all neurons that use GABA are affected in schizophrenia; only one specific type of GABA-containing neuron is affected in the ways mentioned here.[13]

Given that glutamate is excitatory and GABA is inhibitory, it would be tempting to dismiss the effects of their impairments in schizophrenia, if the overall balance between excitation and inhibition remains about the same. But the brain does not work at this scale. Researchers regard the total levels of neurotransmitters as less important than what happens within neural circuits, especially the millions of very small circuits of similar design, called **microcircuits**, which comprise the cerebral cortex. Each microcircuit occupies just a few square micrometers, but together they are responsible for all the basic computing activity in the cortex. They integrate information, generate responses, and contribute to consciousness. All three of the neurotransmitters that have been strongly implicated in schizophrenia—namely, dopamine, glutamate, and GABA—are present in the microcircuits. Although they are found everywhere in the cortex, the microcircuits of the prefrontal cortex have become the focus of research because, as noted earlier, dysfunctions in the prefrontal cortex appear to be responsible for many of the negative symptoms of schizophrenia.

The neuroscientific approach to schizophrenia includes, among other matters, understanding the details of prefrontal lobe microcircuits. These details, beginning with the neurons that constitute the microcircuits and the physiological interactions that occur within them, illustrate just how intricate the human brain is and how difficult it is to remedy its diseases. The key anatomical features of the prefrontal microcircuits, together with a schematic representation of schizophrenia biomarkers, are illustrated in the accompanying figure.

The centerpiece of the cortical microcircuit is the pyramidal cell, so named for its roughly triangular shape. The pyramidal cell is the only cell in the cortical microcircuit that sends messages, in the form of **action potentials**, out from the microcircuit. Whenever an action potential passes down the axon of a pyramidal cell, some piece of information is being transmitted to another region of the brain. Crucially, the pyramidal cell does not fire action potentials at random. It weighs all the excitation and all the inhibition received through its synapses. Only if the *net* excitation exceeds a preset threshold does the cell fire one or more action potentials.

Neuroscientists know an amazing amount of detail about the excitatory and inhibitory inputs to the pyramidal cells. Excitation comes from other pyramidal cells, and it is transmitted by glutamate. Dopamine is also in the picture because it is able to enhance the glutamate effect. If the dopamine-containing cells are active (which depends on

Normal

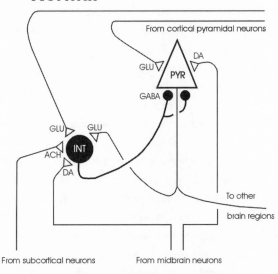

Schizophrenia

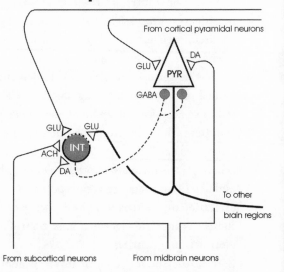

A microcircuit in the prefrontal lobe. In brains of people with schizophrenia, the pyramidal cells are hyperactive due to reduced excitation of inhibitory interneurons and reduced amounts of GABA in inhibitory interneurons. The heavy black lines indicate highly active pathways; the dotted lines and gray markings indicate reduced activity.

the circumstances), the pyramidal cells will become highly excited and will fire many action potentials, thus signaling that the message is urgent or important. Inhibitory signals come to the pyramidal cells from a class of small cells, called **interneurons**, which use GABA as their neurotransmitter.

A biomarker can represent either a cause of symptoms or a consequence of symptoms. In the case of schizophrenia, any abnormal feature in the brain, such as one of the abnormalities illustrated in the figure, could be responsible for creating hallucinations, delusions, or cognitive impairments—hence, it could be a *cause* of the symptoms—or it could be only a *consequence* of medications or lifestyle. Although it is not yet known for certain which of the schizophrenia biomarkers are causative, those in the cortical microcircuits are strong contenders. Specifically, many investigators believe that an impairment of GABA-mediated inhibition accounts for at least some of the symptoms of schizophrenia.

As I have mentioned, brains from people who have schizophrenia contain less GABA and less of the enzyme that makes GABA than do brains from mentally healthy people. Additional evidence for weakened inhibition comes from physiological investigations that show that pyramidal neurons fire more action potentials in the brains of people with schizophrenia than in the brains of people who do not have schizophrenia; this is the inevitable result of reduced inhibition, because firing levels depend on excitation, which is opposed by inhibition. Lastly, a failure of inhibition can be observed in certain behavioral tasks, such as when a research subject is trained to respond to a specific stimulus but also instructed to withhold the response if there is a different stimulus under certain conditions.

For example, a person may be given one second to press a "left" button when a left arrow appears on a screen and a "right" button when a right arrow appears on the screen. If, however, a tone is sounded before the subject presses a button, he or she must not press either button. People with schizophrenia find it difficult to withhold their responses when engaged in this task. Although the failure of behavioral inhibition in this task is intriguing for its resemblance to the loss of physiological inhibition, the most damaging effect of reduced physiological inhibition is likely to be a disruption of basic information processing throughout the prefrontal cortex.

To explore the consequences of impaired inhibition, a group of investigators did a very clever experiment with mice.[14] Using genetic engineering techniques, they introduced a protein into the mouse's prefrontal cortex that caused the pyramidal cells to become hyperactive; thus, the manipulation mimicked the effect of reduced inhibition. Remarkably, the scientists were able to control exactly when the cells were hyperactive by simply directing a bright light to the front part of the brain; they returned the cells to normal levels of activity by turning off the light. The beauty of the technique is that it allowed the investigators to manipulate the pyramidal cells' activity even when the mice were awake and moving around. It was possible, therefore, to compare the animals' behavior under normal conditions and after the pyramidal cells had been rendered hyperactive.

The scientists conducted several tests to determine the effects of cellular hyperactivity on behavior, two of which are of particular interest because they are social in nature. In one, a mouse previously unknown to the experimental animal was dropped into the same cage as the experimental animal. With the light OFF (pyramidal cells working normally), the experimental animal approached the newcomer and repeatedly sniffed and licked him. By contrast, with the light ON (pyramidal cells hyperactive), the experimental animal totally ignored the newcomer. In another test, the experimental mouse was placed in an enclosure that had three "rooms," one of which contained another mouse. With the light OFF, the experimental mouse consistently entered the "social room," but with the light ON, he seldom entered that room. Given that people with schizophrenia typically have social deficits, these results are very interesting, all the more so because they show that prefrontal hyperactivity is the likely *cause* of the behavioral impairments, not merely a side effect of the impairments.

Brain science, like all kinds of science, typically begins with the discovery of an effect and then works backward to identify its cause(s) or mechanism(s). Once scientists identify the cause of an effect, let's call it cause 1, they look for the thing or event that led to cause 1, and call it cause 2; next, they look for the cause of cause 2, and so on. This is known as the *top-down strategy*, and it can continue all the way down to atomic physics. In the example that we have been considering, the effect is schizophrenia symptoms. It has been proposed that one of the responsible mechanisms is hyperactivity in cortical pyramidal cells, which itself can be traced to a partial loss of inhibition in these cells. The next question, therefore, is what causes the reduced inhibition. An answer to this last question could lead to an effective therapy for schizophrenia or perhaps even to its prevention.

There are several possible causes of the weakened inhibition, and all might contribute. I mentioned above that there is less GABA in brains from people with schizophrenia compared to brains from mentally healthy people. Thus, it is possible that the interneurons do not have enough GABA to do a proper job of inhibiting the pyramidal cells. Alternatively, perhaps the interneurons have plenty of GABA but do not get sufficiently excited to release as much of it as is needed. The interneurons receive excitatory signals from three types of neurons using three different neurotransmitters: from cortical pyramidal neurons releasing glutamate, from subcortical neurons releasing acetylcholine, and from neurons in the midbrain releasing dopamine (as shown in the figure). If any of these excitatory inputs is defective, the interneurons will fire fewer than the normal number of action potentials, and, as a result, the pyramidal cells will not be adequately inhibited.

Researchers had good reasons to examine the glutamate input to the interneurons. First, they knew that drugs that antagonize glutamate produce schizophrenia-like symptoms in humans (as mentioned above); second, postmortem analyses had shown that brains from people with schizophrenia contain fewer receptor molecules for glutamate than do brains from people who do not have schizophrenia; and, third, the glutamate signals are part of a feedback loop from pyramidal cell to interneuron to pyramidal cell. Therefore, a group of scientists used genetic engineering to create mice that would lose about 50 percent of their glutamate receptors during early postnatal development.[15]

As predicted, the interneurons were much less sensitive to glutamate in these animals than in normal mice and also less active—hence, less influential in inhibiting pyramidal neurons. Strikingly, the mice displayed several abnormalities that bear a resemblance to schizophrenia, namely, anxiety-like behaviors, memory deficits, heightened startle responses, and a reduced desire for sweet foods. In addition, the investigators demonstrated that the physiological and behavioral effects were evident if the genes were manipulated *before* the mice had fully matured, but not if they were manipulated *after* maturation. The study confirms that glutamate, an excitatory neurotransmitter, is strongly influential (via its effect on interneurons) in regulating cortical inhibition. Not surprisingly, investigators are now looking for a drug or a genetic manipulation that can selectively restore the glutamate receptors on cortical interneurons. If such a drug was safe for use in humans, it could reduce some of the symptoms of schizophrenia.

If I have persuaded you that the microcircuits of the prefrontal cortex are a complex business, I have accomplished my purpose. Even the simplified discussion above suggests that several mechanisms act together to cause microcircuit dysfunction in schizophrenia. The microcircuits do not hold all the answers to the schizophrenia puzzle, but they probably are involved because, in healthy brains, they serve such vital cognitive tasks as short-term memory,[16] attention, planning, and judgment. The ultimate goal of schizophrenia research is to learn how genes, the environment, and the brain all converge to produce observable symptoms. A key part of this effort is to understand how mutated genes disrupt microcircuit functions, as we are reminded by one team of leading researchers:

> The goal of systems biology is to understand how genes work together in biochemical and cellular networks to produce function. Such an integrated understanding is of special importance in schizophrenia research because the disorder results from the synergistic interaction of many risk genes, none of which has a large effect. To determine whether genes act synergistically, it is necessary to have a circuit-based model.[17]

SUMMARY

- The term *mental illness* is misleading because it invites one to imagine an illness of the mind. In fact, mental illness is not in the mind; it is in the brain.
- Biomarkers of schizophrenia include anatomical, physiological, and neurochemical abnormalities, among them thinner cerebral corti-

ces, larger fluid-filled spaces, displaced or absent neurons, and alterations in several of the major neurotransmitter systems (glutamate, gamma-aminobutyric acid, and dopamine).

- One or more of the biomarkers may eventually serve as physical criteria for diagnosis, thereby replacing the psychiatrists' judgments of behavior, which are currently used. However, to be useful in the development of therapeutic agents, alterations that cause the symptoms must be distinguished from alterations that are simply secondary effects, such as from changes in medication and lifestyle.

- Researchers are focusing on the prefrontal cortex because it mediates many of the cognitive functions that fail in schizophrenia. Studies find a weakening of inhibition in microcircuits, which causes a key cell type to fire action potentials at inappropriately high frequencies. Also, electrical events in the prefrontal lobe and the hippocampus are partially disconnected in schizophrenia owing to structural defects in axonal pathways.

- An impairment of glutamate neurotransmission seems to underlie the dysfunction in prefrontal microcircuits. More broadly, genetic evidence and the abundance of biomarkers suggest that schizophrenia is the result of multiple neurodevelopmental errors that act together to impair brain circuits.

13

The Villa and the Ambassador

Jim's experiment with independent living—in Ventura, Santa Monica, and Hollywood—coincided with a broader social experiment, known as *deinstitutionalization*. Thomas Szasz and his fellow antipsychiatrists were arguing that mental illness is but a myth, psychiatric patients are only deviant, and the institutions that house them are primarily institutions of social repression. Meanwhile, mental hospitals were costing taxpayers lots of money, and reports commissioned by Presidents Kennedy and Carter advocated building "therapeutic communities" outside of hospitals. With the new antipsychotic drugs proving effective, the stage was set for releasing patients into local communities where they could be looked after by outpatient services.

The transfer of patients from hospitals to the community began slowly but accelerated when politicians began to act. In 1957 the California legislature passed the Short-Doyle Act (later incorporated into Medi-Cal), which directed funds to cities and counties for community mental health services and gave local officials authority over hospital admissions. The pace of deinstitutionalization in all states increased dramatically after federal legislation established Medicare and Medicaid in 1965 and Supplemental Security Income in 1974, because now states were able to draw upon federal funds to finance their programs. As a result of deinstitutionalization, the number of severely ill mental patients in California's public hospitals declined from 37,318 in 1955 to 9,814 in 1994. If we take into account the very large increase in the total population of California over the same period, the number of severely ill mental patients declined by 95.8 percent, meaning that for every 100 patients hospitalized in 1955, only 4 remained hospitalized in 1994.[1]

Thus, in 1980, when it became apparent that Jim could not live on his own, no one expected him to go back to a hospital. Instead, he moved into to a board-and-care home near the urban center of Los Angeles, where he remained until 1991.

The Portland Villa, as my brother's home was known, was located on Portland Street, but it was hardly a villa. Most of the residents in the immediate neighborhood were recent immigrants from Korea. Just a few blocks away, stood the campus of the University of Southern California, and beyond that loomed the imposing Los Angeles Coliseum. The Villa was a white stucco building that looked much like the other apartment buildings in the area except for the few pretentious embellishments which, in the mind of Mrs. Nelson, validated the appellation *Villa*. Mrs. Nelson was the owner and hands-on manager. She gave Christmas gifts to the residents, and Jim liked her, but throughout her long association with Jim she remained somewhat of a shadowy enigma. Starting with the Villa, Mrs. Nelson progressively expanded her holdings, eventually owning four board-and-care homes. As her stable of facilities increased in size, so too must her fortune have grown, since the state of California paid the residents' fees and there was plenty of money to be made by cutting costs.

Jim lived in all four of those homes, and although I visited him in each of them, I saw Mrs. Nelson only once in 30 years. Toward the end of Jim's life, after he had suffered a major medical event, he was moved to a board-and-care facility run by a different owner. I was astonished to learn that someone phoned Jim's doctor shortly after this move claiming to be his sister (he had none) and demanding that Jim be moved back to Mrs. Nelson's residence. My intervention prevented this, but I was never able to determine whether the imposter was acting on behalf of Mrs. Nelson's compassionate interests or, more likely, seeking to maximize her monetary gains.

It was always difficult to find a parking place near the Villa, but I was lucky on my first visit. The door of the Villa was unlocked, and I stepped into a lounge where several people milled about smoking cigarettes. Then I spotted Jim walking toward me with a broad smile.

"Welcome to the Villa!" he proclaimed.

"Thanks, Jim. It's good to see you."

"I gather you've come by yourself this time. How is the family back in Montreal? What are Zanna and Aaron doing these days?" Jim was quite fond of my daughter, Zanna, and my son, Aaron. He enjoyed their company, and during his one visit to my home in Montreal, he had interacted well with them.

"Everyone is busy. Both kids are in school, of course, and performing well. You may recall that Zanna is learning to play the cello. She likes it a lot and is getting pretty good. We've been trying to interest Aaron in hockey, but so far he's not excited about it. Neither am I, to tell you the truth. It's a drag carrying all his gear down to the arena, and the air inside that place is absolutely stifling."

Just then, a thin, older man approached us. Jim turned to him and introduced me. "Stan, I'd like you to meet my brother, Ron."

"You've got a nice room here," I said, gesturing to several areas evidently devoted to leisure activities. I spotted paint materials, board games, a television set, and bookshelves. A piano with open music sheets stood at the side wall. "It looks like a good place to relax in."

Jim must have sensed my discomfort because, instead of showing me in more detail what the lounge had to offer, he invited me to see his personal room. He led me upstairs to a small room off a central corridor. I was surprised to see everything clean and tidy. I recognized several individual items from our home in Westwood, including a lamp and a mirror. "This looks very comfortable, Jim." Indeed, he would never again have such good accommodations in any establishment run by Mrs. Nelson—or, for that matter, anywhere else.

"It's okay," he said. He noticed that I was looking at his stack of books. "I'm reading *A Single Man*, by Christopher Isherwood. He's a fine English novelist and a good guy, although he is a homosexual. He gave a couple of lectures in one of my classes at UCLA." He paused, and then in a lower tone of voice, "I should speak more softly when I mention UCLA around here—the campus of our enemy, the dreaded USC, is just down the street!"

I sat in a chair while Jim sat on his bed, and we chatted about books, the Villa, and the approaching football season. Jim felt secure at the

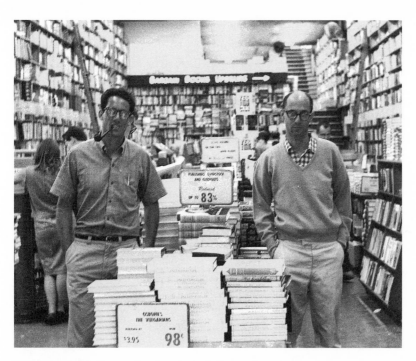

The author and Jim at a bookstore in Hollywood, 1962

Villa. He had friends in the home, some intellectual stimulation from a literary program run by the visiting social worker, and his medication was working as intended. All things considered, it was probably the most stable period in his life. Dad continued to hope for better, but Mom and I were happy enough that he was no longer in a hospital. I saw Jim fairly frequently when I returned to Los Angeles on holidays and in the summer. Jim and I had common interests, mutual respect, and a shared pleasure in being in each other's company. On my initial visit to the Villa we simply took a short walk around the neighborhood, but on every subsequent visit I took Jim somewhere in the car. Often, we would go back to Westwood Village to be with Mom and Dad. On other occasions we would head for Hollywood, where Jim liked browsing in the bookshops. He and I both enjoyed taking lunch at Canter's Deli on North Fairfax Avenue, where we invariably ordered matzo ball soup, hot pastrami sandwiches, and dill pickles.

One time, when I asked Jim where he'd like me to drive him, he replied without hesitation, "I want to go to the Ambassador Hotel." He could see the bewildered look on my face, so he explained that he often went to the Ambassador on his own by taking a public bus. He was no doubt drawn to the hotel by its illustrious history, its lush grounds, and its architectural splendor. There was also the fact that our family had spent a week or two at a more modest hotel close to the Ambassador when we had first arrived in Los Angeles back in 1948. As for the Ambassador, it gained a lasting place in history as the location where Robert Kennedy was assassinated in 1968. (The building was demolished in 2005.)

Driving slowly as we approached the hotel via its long and curvaceous driveway, we passed through a spectacle of water fountains, palm trees, and birds of paradise plants. Inside, as I gawked at the rich furnishings, I sensed that Jim was ill at ease.

"What do you do when you come here?" I asked.

"Oh, I usually just hang out in the lobby. It's quite something isn't it?"

It was indeed beautiful. I noticed the people, too: the well-dressed guests, bedazzled tourists, and uniformed hotel personnel. It occurred to me that Jim was not meant to be in this picture. He was not well dressed, not comfortable in his body, and not at all "cool." His medication had begun to stiffen his movements and bend his posture, so his gangly stature was exaggerated. When he came here by himself, I thought, he must have been the target of many furtive looks as he brooded and fidgeted. Just then Jim started walking unusually fast toward the dining area. I followed him, and when I saw him glance toward the reception desk, I too turned around to look. The clerk at the desk was staring directly at us with stern eyes. Ah, yes, it suddenly occurred to me what was going on. Jim must have had previous run-ins with the hotel management. He probably had not committed any real offense, but his mere presence in this hotel would surely have been unsettling to some people. On this day, he must have brought me along to protect him and comfort him as he tried one more time to visit a place where he knew he was not welcome. I might have been willing to assume these duties, but at the moment, I was no longer enjoying our visit to the Ambassador Hotel.

"Jim," I said as calmly as I could. "I think it's time for us to go."

"Okay," he agreed.

We had to pass the reception desk again on our way out, but we did not look that way. We walked straight across the lobby keeping our eyes squarely on the exit door. From the safety of our car, as we traveled down the hotel driveway with its colorful plant borders, I cautiously offered Jim a word of advice. "You know," I said, "it would probably be better if you found somewhere else to hang out."

Although nothing of substance occurred in the Ambassador Hotel that day, the experience worked its effects on my consciousness. I realized that I had been embarrassed by what had happened, even by what had *not* happened. I had feared a real incident, a guest staring rudely at us, or, worse, someone from the hotel asking us to leave. But what stuck in my mind afterward was simply the embarrassment of being associated with someone—my brother!—who looked and behaved unlike everyone else. People must have recognized that he was mentally ill. And me, a physically fit, smartly dressed, university professor. What was I doing accompanying this misfit? It shames me now to recall these feelings, but I cannot deny them.

Events like those at the Ambassador forced me to accept that my brother was *a schizophrenic*. Today, as I stated earlier, we correctly say that someone "has schizophrenia" or that he or she is a person "with schizophrenia," but in the past, "schizophrenia" stood as a sufficient description of the person. Hence the ugly phrase, Jim *is* a schizophrenic. I abhorred the idea and I resisted it, as did my parents. Mom always said that Jim was "mentally ill," and Dad preferred to speak of "problems" that would eventually disappear. The word *schizophrenia* was not spoken in our family's conversations. In fact, it was only because of my university experience that I was able to put two and two together and conclude that my brother had schizophrenia; after all, my major subject was psychology. Outside of the university, mental illness was generally absent from public discourse, and schizophrenia in particular was almost a dirty word. The subject of schizophrenia was not likely to come up in polite conversations, and people with mental illness were shunned. They were avoided. Just three years before Jim developed psychosis, a pioneering investigator of mental illness stigma wrote:

Mental illness is a very threatening, fearful thing and not an idea to be entertained lightly about anyone. Emotionally, it represents to people a loss of what they consider to be the distinctively human qualities of rationality and free will, and there is a kind of a horror in dehumanization. . . . mental illness is something that people want to keep as far from themselves as possible.[2]

Attitudes such as this explain why few of my friends, colleagues, and relatives knew that Jim was ill, and why none of them knew that he had schizophrenia. I spoke so little about Jim to my best friend, Eugene, that he once referred to me as an only child. We both laughed at his understandable error, but in truth, I, too, was a victim of Jim's stigma. I tried to avoid embarrassment by remaining silent about my brother and by shielding the two of us from being seen in public places.

Why Is Schizophrenia Stigmatized?

In ancient Greece, tattoos were called stigmas. Today, the word *stigma* refers not to a physical mark but to a mark on one's character or reputation. Many individuals who carry the stigma of mental illness suffer from blocked opportunities for employment, terminated friendships, disrupted marriages, and frustration in virtually every life goal that is reliant on social interactions. The stigma of mental illness can also keep people from seeking professional help for their mental illnesses. Studies in the United States estimate that "nearly two-thirds of all people with diagnosable mental disorders [real disorders] do not seek treatment."[1] A survey conducted for the Canadian Medical Association found that only 50 percent of respondents would tell their friends or co-workers that they have a family member with mental illness, compared to 72 percent for diagnoses of cancer and 68 percent for diabetes.[2] Only 46 percent of respondents in a U.S. survey said they would tell friends that they had been treated for schizophrenia.[3] Clearly, attitudes such as these have profound effects on people with schizophrenia. We must ask, then, what causes stigma and what can be done about it?

It is widely believed that the association of mental illness with violence creates stigma. The news media and the entertainment industry perpetuate the stereotype of the violent mentally ill person by exploiting sensational cases. This focus increases readership and viewer ratings but it misleads the public. In reality, people with mental illness commit violent acts only slightly more often than do mentally healthy people, and in almost all cases it is when they are abusing drugs or are dependent on drugs. Two leading researchers conducted a survey of

34,653 individuals in the United States, collecting data on the persons' mental health and participation, if any, in substance abuse, drug dependency, and violence. After analyzing the results, the investigators wrote:

> Such data are at odds with public fears such as those reported in a national survey in which 75 percent of the sample viewed people with mental illness as dangerous and 60 percent believed people with schizophrenia were likely to commit violent acts. Instead, the current results show that if a person has severe mental illness *without substance abuse and history of violence*, he or she has the same chances of being violent during the next 3 years as any other person in the general population [emphasis mine].[4]

In my opinion, the stigma of mental illness goes deeper than the fear of violence. I think it has more to do with people's gut reactions, their implicit understanding of the nature of mental illness. At the root of stigma lies the assumption that people with mental illness are themselves responsible for their diseases. The public stigmatizes them because they are seen to be morally tainted and because they seem unwilling to overcome their illnesses. My views about this are unconventional, so let me explain.

All of us carry a set of basic philosophical assumptions that influence our perceptions. Fundamental to our perception of mental illness are assumptions about the mind and its relationship to the body. For the most part, these are unstated and unquestioned assumptions. For these reasons, it can be difficult to know exactly what people think about mind-body issues, but there are good grounds for concluding that most people are philosophical dualists—in other words, they believe that the mind and the body are two separate "things."[5] It is interesting to read the opinion of no less of an authority than the Office of the United States Surgeon General: "Explanations for stigma stem, in part, from the misguided split between mind and body first proposed by Descartes."[6] For dualists, as I have already argued, mental illness is literally *in the mind*. Whereas Descartes wrote of the mind only as the agent of rational thinking, others can readily imagine a disordered and irrational mind. Importantly, too, Descartes insisted that the mind is completely free; it governs the brain and initiates human actions. This is what Descartes wrote about free will in his *Meditations*,

> It is free-will alone or liberty of choice which I find to be so great in me that I can conceive no other idea to be more great; it is indeed the case that it is for the most part this will that causes me to know that in some manner I bear the image and similitude of God. For although the power of will is incomparably greater in God than in me . . . , it nevertheless does not seem to me greater if I consider it formally and precisely in itself.[7]

Descartes, a devout Catholic and an admirer of the theologian Saint Thomas Aquinas, took from Aquinas his notions of the soul and free will. Both men believed that the human body is machine-like, as it is in animals, but that the soul is unique to humans. They equated the soul and the mind, and they said that this "thing" is the essence of human life. Although Descartes exalts the freedom of the mind/soul in the passage quoted above, there is a downside to freedom, and that is personal responsibility, as Aquinas stressed. I believe that the stigma of mental illness derives from the exaggerated notion of personal responsibility that springs from a dualistic philosophy. My argument will continue after a brief review of relevant history.

Before mental illness became a special kind of illness, there were only illnesses, all of which were presumed to be physical. Hippocrates believed that madness was caused by problems in the body,[8] but most of his contemporaries did not consider madness an illness. Rather, they thought that it was caused by the actions of gods. Later, in medieval times, people blamed madness on the evil influences of an assortment of entities that included devils, witches, succubae, incubi, and werewolves. People who exhibited irrational or uncontrollable behaviors were sent away to special holding centers known as asylums. The conditions in these asylums were generally abysmal, and there were no effective treatments.

Early in the nineteenth century, two influential reformers appeared on the scene, William Tuke in England and Philippe Pinel in France. Although the two men arrived with very different backgrounds, they had both come to the conclusion that their patients suffered from some type of psychological defect, and they felt that the patients would respond better to kindness and religious observance than to punishment and neglect. Tuke and Pinel independently introduced practices that encouraged their patients to voluntarily adopt a well-ordered, moderate lifestyle. The English called the program *moral therapy* because it was centered on the doctors' ability to foster good behavior in their patients. With the apparent success of moral therapy, more and more people began to believe that the patients, previously referred to as *mad*, were actually suffering from a special type of illness, a disease of the mind or *mental illness*. Later, when highly trained anatomists failed to find anything unusual in the brains of deceased patients, this was seen as additional evidence of a purely mental illness.[9] Thereafter, people sought to understand the nonphysical cause of the newly designated nonphysical illnesses.

It was only natural that people would look to the mind for the cause of mental illness, especially given that the mind was supposed to be completely free. From these origins came the notion that people with schizophrenia are to be blamed for their own disease. Bernard Weiner is a social psychologist who has studied the roots of the blaming process.[10] He documented the nearly universal human tendency to assign personal responsibility for things that go wrong, and he showed that such assignments lead directly to moral blame and anger directed toward the responsible individual. Putting all of this together, I believe that the stigma of schizophrenia can be explained, at least in part, by the entangled ideas of dualism, free will, personal responsibility, and moral blame. A similar view has been expressed by a philosopher of medicine who wrote, "The puzzle about mental illness is that it seems to be an activity of the very seat of responsibility—the mind and character—and therefore to be beyond all hope of excuse."[11]

The belief that people with mental illnesses are responsible for their diseases is widespread. Evidence for this conclusion comes from several large, well-designed surveys of public opinion. In one survey, conducted in the United States, people were presented with descriptions of fictitious individuals who had experienced symptoms that were typical of one or another mental illness. When asked what they thought were the causes of the symptoms representative of schizophrenia, 33 percent chose the person's "own bad character."[12]

A German survey used similar methods. The participants read short stories describing behaviors typical of schizophrenia, and then they were asked to indicate the cause or causes. A stunning 50 percent of respondents cited "lack of will power" as a cause of schizophrenia.[13] Lastly, in 2008 the Canadian Medical Association conducted a major survey of public opinion concerning mental illness. A significant minority of respondents, 10 percent, agreed with the statement, "Most people with mental illnesses could just snap out of it if they really wanted to."[14] In summary, these polls reveal a particular type of ignorance about schizophrenia and other mental disorders. They indicate a readiness to hold the victims personally responsible for their illnesses.

The idea that mental patients can resolve their own problems is not new. The moral therapies of the early nineteenth century, for example, were built on the very same notion. Physicians acting under the leadership of either William Tuke or Philippe Pinel mixed mild punishments with kindly persuasion in trying to motivate patients toward more normal patterns of behavior. Similarly, some caregivers today reason that if a mental illness is caused by acts (or omissions) of free will, then other willful acts (or omissions) might undo the illness.

In the movie *A Beautiful Mind*, the Nobel laureate John Nash is shown reasoning his way out of his psychosis. He, however, is unique in many respects, most notably because of his exceptional intelligence. Despite these advantages, he struggled for three decades before emerging from schizophrenia. For most other individuals suffering from schizophrenia, no amount of thinking will alleviate the symptoms. Whereas dualistic thinking fosters optimistic ideas like "mind over matter," reality suggests that to encourage self-healing is to raise false hopes and invite disappointments.

The emotionally charged ideas of free will and moral responsibility also figure in the shameful treatment of mentally disturbed persons. Throughout history, mentally ill people were commonly, and sometimes severely, mistreated. In the Middle Ages, "mad men" and "mad women" were chained to trees, beaten, and even burned to death as punishments for their perceived sins. Even in modern times, stories of abuse occasionally come to light, and all too often patients with mental illnesses are treated disrespectfully in psychiatric facilities. I think it is reasonable to conclude that moral attitudes lie behind such mistreatments. People may consider it acceptable to mistreat a patient if they view that person as having neither the "sense" nor the "character" to act normally.

What can be done about mental illness stigma? We must start with an effective educational campaign that emphasizes two points. First, to counter the perception that people with mental illnesses are prone to acts of violence, the facts, as summarized above, need to be emphasized over and over again. Second, the neurobiological basis of mental disorders must be presented in enough detail to demonstrate that schizophrenia and similar disorders are in the brain, not in the mind. Instead of referring to these disorders as *mental* illnesses, we should adopt a term that better reflects their physical nature. But changing the vocabulary will not be easy. I regret that, despite my convictions, I have not been able to write this book without repeatedly using the term *mental illness*. I considered writing *so-called mental illness*, but this is clumsy, and the preferred alternatives, *brain disorder* and *neuropsychiatric illness*, are still too unfamiliar. I conclude that we should probably wait until the public's understanding of psychiatric science is updated before we worry about changing terminology.

Several organizations that advocate on behalf of the mentally ill have attempted to portray mental illness as a brain disorder. For example, the group known as NAMI declares, "Just as diabetes is a disorder of the pancreas, mental illnesses are medical conditions." It further states, "Schizophrenia is a disorder of the brain, caused by problems with brain chemistry and brain structure." Unfortunately, the message sent by NAMI is contradicted by its own name, the National Alliance on Mental Illness. Organizations such as NAMI deserve credit for educating the public on the nature of mental illnesses, but their arguments have had little or no impact on popular language usage.

Even more disconcerting than the resistance to new terminology is evidence that the campaigns portraying mental illnesses as brain illnesses have, so far, not moved public opinion. On the contrary, surveys in the United States, Germany, and elsewhere indicate that while factual knowledge of mental illnesses has increased, so too have attitudes attributed to stigma increased. For example, one U.S. study compared data from two large surveys conducted 10 years apart. After reporting the results, the authors concluded that

> in surveys from both 1996 and 2006 . . . holding a neurobiological conception of mental illness either was unrelated to stigma or tended to increase the odds of a stigmatizing reaction. Our most striking finding is that stigma among the American public appears to be surprisingly fixed, even in the face of . . . advances in public knowledge.[15]

Why are these campaigns not working as intended? Leaving aside the possibility that the publicity is poorly designed or inadequately distributed, I suggest that the problem lies in the philosophical assumptions to which I referred above. The authors of the campaigns want people to understand that there are biological explanations for mental illness. They tell people that if there are valid physical causes (genes, neurons, neurotransmitters), then no individual should be blamed for his or her own illness, and no stigma should be applied. This makes sense to me because I believe in a **monist** philosophy of mind in which the mind is nothing but an aspect of the brain's physiological activity.

A dualist, however, is likely to think differently. I suspect that a dualist will accept, as an intellectual fact, that mental illnesses have biological causes while continuing to believe, from intuition alone, that mental illnesses are voluntary. Dualism makes it possible to hold both beliefs, because it claims two levels of control over human behavior: first, the mind controls the brain; and, second, the brain controls behavior. Thus, people may say that the mechanical, or physical, cause of mental illness lies in the brain, but the ultimate cause is in the mind. I can imagine a dualist acknowledging that the brain is subject to scientific scrutiny while at the same time proclaiming that the hyperactivity of pyramidal cells in the prefrontal lobe is caused by mental events that are independent of any physical thing. For me, such an explanation makes no sense.

SUMMARY

- Persons with schizophrenia carry the burden of a stigma that stymies their social lives, blocks their chances for employment, and interferes with treatments.

- Although a fear of violence may contribute to creating stigma, studies show that mentally ill individuals are, in fact, no more violent than other citizens, except when they also abuse drugs or have drug dependencies. When the media call attention to sensational cases, the stories fuel stigma.

- People who tacitly believe in philosophical dualism are likely to believe that mental illness is, literally, in the mind. This leads them to conclude that the victim of mental illness is himself or herself responsible for the disease. In public opinion surveys, many people cite "lack of will power" and "bad character" as causes of schizophrenia. Attitudes such as these contribute to stigma by assigning blame.

- The frequent mistreatment of people with mental illness can be understood as punishment for what is perceived as a weak will or a corrupted soul.

- Educational campaigns need to address three issues. First, misconceptions about the likelihood of violence must be corrected. Second, education on neuroscience must be intensified so that the physical basis of mental illness becomes obvious. Third, and most daunting, people need to be persuaded that philosophical dualism is wrongheaded; in reality, the world contains only physical things.

- The term *mental illness* will eventually be abandoned in favor of an alternative term that recognizes the physical basis of behavioral and psychological disorders.

15

Strolling the Boardwalk at Hermosa Beach

We were never sure what to expect when we visited my brother. He could be calm and pleasant, he could be agitated, or he could be sullen. On this occasion, we were relieved to see him approach us with a beaming smile. "Hi, Ron," he said, "Welcome to the retirement home." And then, in a lower voice, "Hi, Dad." Mom had died a few years earlier, so it was just Dad and me on this visit. Jim led us into the sunny courtyard of the Centinela Retirement Home, where we found a dozen or more residents scattered around.

Jim had moved to the Centinela Retirement Home from the Portland Villa following a period of psychotic instability, some weeks of which he had spent in a psychiatric hospital. The Retirement Home was located in Inglewood conveniently close to Orange County where our parents had moved after *their* retirement. However, this was by no means an ordinary retirement home. It was, in fact, just another psychiatric board-and-care facility, but for people slightly older than the residents of the Portland Villa. The ironic name, like that of the Villa, was invented by the owner, Mrs. Nelson. By the time I visited the Retirement Home with Dad, I had already been there once or twice by myself. I had also learned to recognize it from the air as I flew into Los Angeles from Montreal, which was *my* new home. The Centinela Retirement Home was easy to spot because it was situated very close to the Hollywood Park horse racetrack. From the air, the distinctive racing oval and the huge parking lot were unmistakable. As the plane descended toward the airport, I located Hollywood Park and then spotted the Retirement Home just before we swept past its rooftop.

Seen from the ground, the establishment blended in well with the single-family homes and apartment buildings of the working-class neighborhood. Its architectural style was vaguely Spanish, owing to the courtyard, the red stucco roof, and the potted palms. Three single-story buildings surrounded the courtyard; one contained rooms for the residents, one was an office, and the third combined a dining area and a television lounge. The television area was set up like a small theater and suitably darkened. A grouping of chairs was positioned in front of, and beneath, the television which hung suspended from the ceiling at a height unreachable by even the tallest resident. Thus, the half-dozen residents who seemed to be perpetually seated in front of the screen were captives to whatever program happened to be on.

Dad and I were still adjusting to the scene in the courtyard, with residents milling about, when Jim asked, "Would you like to meet my new roommate?" Jim had previously mentioned his roommate, Don, who was rumored to be a sports enthusiast. Evidently, he and Jim were quite friendly, so we were anxious to meet him. We followed Jim down a row of doors until we reached his room. The arrangement resembled a motel, so much so that I suspect Centinela had originally functioned as a motel.

Jim proudly announced our presence, "Don," he said, "I'd like you to meet my father, Joe, and my brother, Ron."

"Nice to meet you," replied Don. "I was just going out for a smoke. I hope you enjoy your time together." And with that, he was gone.

"Don's a good guy," offered Jim. "He likes sports. Yesterday the Dodgers were victorious over the Giants. Fernando Valenzuela was pitching. He improved his record to 15 and 6. Dusty Baker came through with a clutch home run to win the game. Now L.A. has won its last four games against San Francisco. They play the Padres next."

Their room was tiny: two beds separated by no more than two feet, a night table beside each bed, and one very small chest of drawers. There was no closet and barely enough space for the three of us to move around. Don's side of the room was cluttered with gadgets, clothing, and pictures of his sporting heroes. His radio was tuned to an all-sports station, and Jim said that it was always on. By contrast, Jim's side was extraordinarily neat.

I noticed a couple of books on Jim's night table. One, I recall, was *Letting Go*, Philip Roth's first novel, published in 1962. Jim often mentioned this book as one of his favorites; he once told me that it was his ambition to write in the style of Philip Roth. However, when I asked whether he was rereading it, he simply replied, "No, I'm not reading anything now."

"What about writing, Jim? Remember, we talked about writing up some of your experiences at the Villa and here at the Retirement Home. You agreed that some of your co-residents were interesting and that there were stories to be told. How is it going? Have you written anything?"

"I started something, but it's not very good. I don't know what I did with those papers, but it doesn't matter. I don't feel like writing."

Dad had been looking around, and now he seemed upset. "Tell me, Jim, where is that nice clock radio that your mother and I gave you for your birthday?"

"Oh, it disappeared. Maybe somebody took it."

"Did you look for it? Did you speak with someone in the office?"

"No."

Evidently the radio had met the same fate as the handsome knitted sweater that Mom had given him one Christmas; it too had "disappeared" within a short time. (We blended Christmas and Hanukkah into a single gift-giving holiday.)

Although Dad and I saw Jim's room as tiny and dreary, Jim seemed pleased with his accommodation. For the time being (it wouldn't last), he was enjoying the company of his peculiar but outgoing roommate, and he felt secure. I took note of Jim's positive mood, and I myself felt buoyed by the Southern California sunshine, so I ventured a suggestion, "What do you say we go to Hermosa Beach?" Jim gave his approval, Dad nodded his consent, and off we went.

We drove south on the Pacific Coast Highway. Hermosa Beach is, or was, a small, friendly, unassuming town. In the late 1950s my friends and I would occasionally drive down from Westwood Village on a Sunday afternoon to hear jazz at a bar called the Lighthouse. We sipped soft drinks and listened to our heroes Shorty Rogers, Bud Shank, and Shelly Manne, along with other "West Coast" musicians. Another great feature in the area is the boardwalk, called the Strand, which lies between the wide, sandy beach and the town. The three of us walked at a slow pace from our parking spot to the boardwalk. Soon our stroll brought us to the intersection of the boardwalk and Pier Avenue. We had arrived at the epicenter of Hermosa Beach.

We moved aside as people of all ages and all physical shapes passed by in four directions. There was a good racial mix and a good locomotion mix: some people were on bicycles or skateboards, others jogged, and the rest were walking. Most wore beach clothing, but there were also a few business types who were obviously on a lunch break, and several others who wore practically nothing at all. We stopped to take in the scene. While Jim and Dad rested on a bench, my attention was drawn to a bearded man standing behind a small table and speaking in a public voice. It turned out that he was pushing a petition to prohibit affirmative action programs at California universities; in essence, these programs established lower admissions standards for blacks than for Caucasians. I argued briefly with the man, and then walked away without signing the petition. When I told Dad and Jim about my encounter with the petitioner, Dad did not hesitate in announcing his support for affirmative action. "It's the right thing to do to correct a historical injustice," he said. Jim kept quiet until I encouraged him to speak his mind.

"The United States has a long history of racial conflict. Abraham Lincoln, Dad's hero, was a champion of the Negro. The Union's victory in the Civil War was supposed to put an end to racial discrimination, but it did not. Now blacks want to go to universities, and I think they should be allowed to go. It's a big issue right now . . . some people are in favor of it, while others are against it."

"Yes, Jim," I asked impatiently, "but do *you* support affirmative action?"

"It's a complex issue. If Dad is for it, then so am I."

His statement on affirmative action was typical. At this stage in the progression of his disease, he no longer spoke at length on any subject, and his conversation tended to be abstract. On occasions like this, when others would be inclined to relate their personal experiences or express their personal beliefs, my brother pronounced as if he were delivering a canned academic summary.

The walking had made us hungry, so we opted to buy chili dogs from a cart. After loading up with French fries, and pouring mustard and relish over the dogs, we walked onto the pier cradling our baskets of food. We chose a bench that allowed us to watch the fishers whose rods stood at attention on the far side of the pier. Seagulls swooped and dove after every scrap of dropped food or bait. While we ate, an assortment of characters came and went in front of us. After one particularly colorful fellow passed by, Jim joked, "He's probably taking a break from his job at the circus." After lunch, with the blazing sun beginning to take its toll, we decided to head back to Inglewood.

Returning to the car by way of Pier Avenue, we came upon The Lighthouse, which was open. I took a peek inside. The interior looked much different than I remembered it from 25 years earlier, but the sight of the stage brought back a flood of nostalgic memories.

"You like jazz, don't you, Ron?"

"Yes, Jim, I certainly *did*. I still listen to it occasionally but not so much as before. Remember when I'd come down here with my friends, Lee and Bob? Bob played the drums, Lee played the trombone, and I played alto sax. There was another kid who imitated Chet Baker on the trumpet. We were all big jazz fans."

Jim made a further attempt at conversation, but what came out was another of his academic discourses. "Jazz is the only truly American contribution to music. It is an art form created by Negroes. The slaves that came to America from West Africa sang while they worked. It helped them to survive hardships. Jazz music as we know it today began in the early part of the twentieth century when Dixieland groups started up in New Orleans. Later, Igor Stravinsky used jazz themes in some of his compositions, for example, in the Ebony Concerto. Of course, George Gershwin was also heavily influenced by Negro jazz, and Aaron Copland and Leonard Bernstein, too. Jazz has made important contributions to serious music."

"But . . . you don't like it, do you?"

"Well, it's all right, but it was more your kind of music, Ron."

Usually after an outing like this, Jim would be tired and exceptionally quiet, sometimes irritable as well. On this day, however, he was still strong as we drove back to Inglewood from Hermosa Beach. He surprised

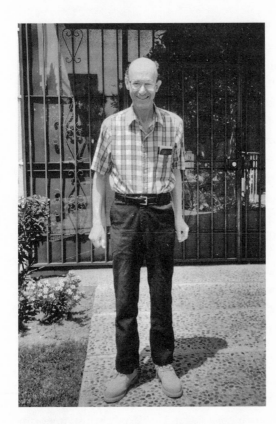

Jim at the Centinela Retirement Home in Inglewood. He is wearing his new pair of shoes.

Dad and me by announcing that he would like to buy a pair of shoes. This was really something! I could not recall having shopped with him ever before, and he seldom expressed a need for anything. Fortunately, we were driving through an area with strip malls. So we pulled into a mall and headed for the shoe shop. I anticipated a difficult time, what with Dad constantly on edge and me concerned about how Jim might behave interacting with the salesperson. In the event, however, all went remarkably well. The salesman was polite and unassuming. Jim told the man what he wanted, the salesman showed him some styles, and Jim chose the one that he liked best. The two of them then worked to find the right size. Dad was more than happy to pay the bill. I saw Jim proudly wearing the shoes on my next visit, but I never saw them again after that.

Yes, it was a memorable day, probably the most enjoyable visit that I had with Jim during his 13 years at the Centinela Retirement Home. By contrast, on subsequent visits (when I came without Dad), Jim often greeted me with a bent body and a down-turned face. We would pass the time by walking a block or two in his neighborhood, but neither of us said much. Meanwhile, Jim's relationships with his fellow board-and-care residents grew more strained. He even had problems with his roommate, Don. Don had once been a friend with whom Jim could share his interest in sports, but later Don became an annoyance with few, if any, redeeming qualities. There were incidents between the two of them, even physical altercations, and Jim was moved to a different room with a new roommate. However, the new pairing led to a new set of problems and further incidents.

On the whole, Jim's condition was deteriorating. He became more depressed, more irritable, and more prone to irrational acts. I observed these developments mostly from afar because I was living in Montreal, but Dad kept me informed, and Jim sent me an occasional letter. It was evident from the letters that his attitude had turned negative. A revelation in one letter struck me as particularly significant. It concerned a subscription to *Time* magazine, which I had given him earlier, at a time when he seemed to be taking an interest in events outside the walls of the Retirement Home. I asked him, in one of my letters, whether he was still reading *Time*. When he reported, in a matter-of-fact manner, that he never read a word of it, I was crushed. I took it as a sign that he had given up trying to participate, even from afar, in the world of action and accomplishment.

The decline of Jim's spirit was easy to see, but his overall status during these years at the Centinela Retirement Home puzzled me. I knew that he had schizophrenia, but I saw none of the cardinal symptoms of schizophrenia, namely, paranoia, hallucinations, and bizarre behaviors. Yes, there was the occasional dust-up with one or another of the residents, but Jim generally behaved as the reserved intellectual that he was. He could engage a visitor in cordial, even witty, conversations, and for a while at least, he took an interest in world affairs. There was definitely something wrong with him, but I could not pinpoint exactly what it was. I dismissed his extreme sensitivity and awkward mannerisms as parts of an unusual personality, not symptoms of a disease. Nevertheless, it was clear that he had withdrawn from the world in which *I* was living and had entered a far less rich one.

The physical environment of the Centinela Retirement Home was of course very different from the family homes in which he had lived for most of the preceding 25 years, but so too were the impoverished lifestyles and the dulled outlooks that he and his fellow residents had adopted. Gone were the days when we in the family fantasized about his holding down a job and living independently. There were no such dreams in this place. Time and time again, I asked myself how he was able to accept the confines of the Retirement Home. I found the place downright depressing, and I am sure that every other outsider felt the same way about it. However, Jim seldom complained, and when he did, it was about small things like the noise from his roommate's radio. Only now do I understand that much of what I have described can be credited to, or blamed upon, his antipsychotic medications. They worked exactly according to the textbook descriptions. They controlled his positive symptoms (delusions, hallucinations, disorganized thought), but they did little for his negative symptoms (apathy, dulled affect, lack of ambition), which persisted and grew worse.

With time, the drugs began to lose their grip, and Jim became paranoid. As a result, he got involved in more altercations, and there was one troublesome incident in which he verbally abused a member of the staff. Also, he became increasingly depressed and withdrawn. Jim himself came to recognize the unsatisfactory state of his life at the Retirement Home. When Mrs. Nelson offered him the opportunity to move to yet another of her board-and-care facilities, he accepted the offer. Whether the move was initiated by him or by her, I do not know, but we all hoped that a change of environment would bring a renewal of his spirit.

16

Just What Is Schizophrenia, Anyway?

Trying to define schizophrenia is like trying to define democracy. We think we know what the terms mean, but, in fact, different people understand them differently. Whereas most people think that democracy describes the type of political system that is currently in place in many countries around the world, academics think of democracy as an abstract, idealistic concept. Similarly, although most people consider schizophrenia a type of mental illness, some critics think that it is not an illness at all but rather a term designating certain deviant behaviors.

A contentious issue in all of these arguments is what to include in the defining description. For example, while nearly all political scientists say that elections are essential for a democracy, opinions vary as to whether one-party elections are okay and whether elections can be democratic when voting rights are restricted to men, to Caucasians, or to the wealthy. Some commentators believe that freedom of expression is a key requirement for a democratic society, while others say that it is desirable but not essential. One way to resolve the problem is to define democracy not as a single thing, but rather as a type of political system that itself comprises numerous subtypes. One speaks, for example, of parliamentary democracies, presidential democracies, liberal democracies, and direct democracies. In the paragraphs below, I will discuss some of the difficulties of trying to define schizophrenia. As with democracy, the problem can be resolved by defining schizophrenia as a collective term representing a group of related, but distinct, psychiatric disorders.

A telling judgment on the current situation regarding the definition of schizophrenia appears in the opening declaration of a recent scholarly article,

> The last several decades have witnessed a steady accrual of a substantive body of knowledge in schizophrenia. However, the concept of schizophrenia as a disease entity, which has survived for over a century, is still mired in controversy and remains unsatisfactory to researchers and clinicians.[1]

To gain perspective on this statement, we need to review the history of the "concept of schizophrenia as a disease entity." The concept originated in Europe in the second half of the nineteenth century, where the disease in question was initially named **dementia praecox**, or premature dementia. A German doctor, Emil Kraepelin, is credited with coining the term and providing its first description, but other European psychiatrists had similar ideas around the same time. A careful reading of the published works of these men shows that each of them recognized similarities among certain groups of patients, and yet none was confident about how, exactly, to define the disease affecting them. There were borderline cases and other exceptions of one sort or another.

Kraepelin first described dementia praecox in his influential textbook, published in 1893, where he also speculated on its biological causes. Eighteen years later, Eugen Bleuler, a professor of psychiatry in Zurich, published his own textbook in which he gave dementia praecox a new name, schizophrenia, and a new description. In contrast to Kraepelin's emphasis on biology, Bleuler focused on the mental states of his patients. Here, for example, is Bleuler's explanation of how his interpretation of the disorder dictated his choice of terminology,

> I call dementia praecox "schizophrenia" because . . . the "splitting" of the different psychic functions is one of its most important characteristics. . . . If the disease is marked, the personality loses its unity; at different times different psychic complexes seem to represent the personality . . . one set of complexes dominates the personality for a time, while other groups of ideas or drives are "split off" and seem either partly or completely impotent.[2]

Bleuler's emphasis on the disruption, or splitting, of consciousness unfortunately led to the popular notion that schizophrenia involves multiple personalities, which it does not. Nevertheless, his insights were very influential within the psychiatric profession, in large part because his interpretation of schizophrenia formed the basis for its description in the first edition of the *Diagnostic and Statistical Manual of Mental Disorders* (DSM-I). The purpose of DSM-I, published in 1952, was to standardize nomenclature and establish consistent diagnostic procedures. However, its publication sparked numerous controversies, which led to revisions. As a result, Bleuler's broad psychological criteria were buried in subsequent editions (DSM-II and DSM-III), and the burden of diagnosis for schizophrenia has shifted to the more obvious psychotic symptoms of delusions and hallucinations.

The current edition, DSM-5, which was released in May 2013, incorporates diverse criteria for the diagnosis of schizophrenia. Its somewhat cumbersome formulation requires a doctor to confirm three essential clinical findings, from which I quote here in a condensed version with my words added in brackets.

> *First*, evidence of two or more psychotic symptoms from the following list: delusions, hallucinations, disorganized speech, catatonic or severely disorganized behaviors; and negative symptoms, i.e. affective flattening [reduced emotional expressions], alogia [inability to speak], or avolition [lack of motivation]. *Second*, social or occupational dysfunction. *Third*, continuous signs of the disturbance persist[ing] for at least six months.[3]

A similar set of requirements is laid out in the *International Statistical Classification of Diseases and Related Health Problems* (ICD-10), which is the current European equivalent of DSM-5. Although the definitions of *schizophrenia* found in DSM-5 and ICD-10 are widely used by psychiatric professionals, they are seriously flawed, as will become apparent in the paragraphs below.

The important role of diagnostic criteria came to light when psychiatrists realized that the rates of prevalence for schizophrenia were several times higher in the United States than in Britain. Suspecting that the discrepancy might be due to the use of different diagnostic criteria in the two nations, a group of investigators conducted an experiment.[4] At the time of their study, 1971, the American psychiatrists were guided by DSM-II, whereas the British psychiatrists relied on ICD-8. The researchers recruited a large number of psychiatrists from both countries who were asked to view videotaped patient interviews. After watching each interview, the psychiatrists gave their diagnoses. The results showed that, in every case, a greater percentage of the American doctors thought that the patient had schizophrenia than did the British doctors. In certain cases, the discrepancies were extremely large. For example, one patient was diagnosed with schizophrenia by 69 percent of the American doctors, compared to just 2 percent for the British doctors; in a second case, the numbers were 85 percent for the Americans versus 7 percent for the British.

The authors of the study noted that "disagreements as glaring as this have serious implications." As they went on to explain,

> Probably the most important cause of the Anglo-American discrepancies revealed here is that the American concept of schizophrenia has expanded greatly in the last 30 years without any corresponding enlargement of the British concept. The reasons for this divergence are complex, but the greater influence of the psychoanalytic movement in North America . . . [has] probably been more important than any factual discoveries.[5]

In 1980, nine years after publication of these results, a new edition of the American diagnostic manual (DSM-III) appeared in which the definition of schizophrenia was considerably narrowed. Not surprisingly, the number of cases reported in the United States fell thereafter. In fact, by the 1990s the relative frequency of schizophrenia diagnoses had been reversed; now *fewer* patients were being diagnosed with schizophrenia in the United States than in Britain.

A major problem with the current definition of schizophrenia is that it relies on subjective judgments. It requires the psychiatrist to decide, for example, whether the patient's behavior is "severely" disorganized and whether he or she lacks motivation. As a result, when any two observers examine the same data through the lenses of their different perceptions and different biases, there is a good chance that the observers will reach different conclusions. This was especially true for the previous edition, which required that the physician make an all-or-none decision on each item. The symptoms must have been deemed either severe enough to warrant a diagnosis of schizophrenia or not so great as to exceed the normal range, whatever that may be. Some improvement has been made in DSM-5, which now include scales for rating the relative severity of certain symptoms, but the fundamental reliance on subjective criteria remains.

Note also that the DSM-5 criteria allow two individuals with very different symptoms both to be diagnosed with schizophrenia. For example, one person may have only delusions (a positive symptom) and reduced affect (a negative symptom), while another person may have only disorganized speech (a positive symptom) and reduced motivation (a negative symptom). Although both individuals have symptoms that satisfy the *Manual*'s criteria for schizophrenia, their symptoms are dissimilar and do not overlap.

The vagueness of the diagnostic criteria causes psychiatrists to make difficult decisions, and because the diagnoses are based almost entirely on subjective judgments, two physicians can easily deliver different diagnoses for the same patient; scientists refer to such diagnoses as "unreliable." In principle, diagnoses could be made highly reliable if physical tests with objective scores were used instead of subjective judgments. Something like the blood sugar test for diabetes would be ideal. Several of the biomarkers of schizophrenia that were mentioned in chapter 12 could potentially serve as objective tests, but each biomarker currently suffers from one or more weaknesses as a diagnostic tool.

To be effective as a diagnostic tool, a biomarker must be present in all or nearly all persons with schizophrenia while absent in all or nearly all persons without schizophrenia; it must be unmistakably recognizable; it must be obtained without violating patients' rights; and, obviously, postmortem biomarkers will not do. To date, no biomarker satisfies all these requirements, although enlarged brain ventricles and reduced gray matter come close. Unfortunately, a catch-22 also blocks the use of biomarkers in diagnoses. To validate any particular biomarker as a reliable indicator of a particular psychiatric disorder, it must be shown that the biomarker is strongly (i.e., reliably) associated with the disorder. However, it will be difficult to establish a statistically valid association so long as the disorders remain ill-defined and unreliably diagnosed.[6]

The *Manual's* consideration of schizophrenia does not stop with the one vague definition. It goes on to define several other disorders that are closely aligned with schizophrenia, thus following a long disposition in psychiatry for naming and categorizing types of mental illness. In the Middle Ages and earlier, the words *hysteria* and *melancholia* were used to distinguish two kinds of common but minor (neurotic) disorders. Later, psychiatric syndromes came to be named for specific symptoms and circumstances; some examples include "old maid's insanity," "moon madness," "masturbatory insanity," and the French-only *la bouffée délirante*, which translates as "eruptive delusional disorder."

Emil Kraepelin changed all of that with his radically new classification of 1899. He placed all the major disorders for which there was no known biological cause into two big categories, one for disorders that involved disturbed moods, and one for disorders in which moods were unaffected. And then he went further. He coalesced all the mood disorders into "manic-depressive psychosis" (later called bipolar disorder) and all the disorders without mood alterations into "dementia praecox" (later called schizophrenia). Kraepelin's neat scheme greatly simplified matters, but it did not satisfy the demands of practitioners for recognition of certain conditions that resembled schizophrenia but were not exactly schizophrenia. And so, the number of disorders proliferated once again. The current edition of the *Manual* lists, in addition to schizophrenia pure and not-so-simple, several related syndromes, namely schizotypal personality disorder, schizophreniform disorder, schizoaffective disorder, and "psychotic disorder not otherwise specified."

Most of the problems in defining schizophrenia stem from its highly variable symptoms, which lead experts to describe it as a *heterogeneous* disease. There have been attempts to formalize the types of schizophrenia on the basis of its clinical symptoms. The early textbooks of Eugen Bleuler (1911) and Emil Kraepelin (1919) already mentioned four types, namely paranoid, catatonic, hebephrenic, and simple. These same types were still present in DSM-IV, with minor changes and one addition: paranoid, catatonic, disorganized, undifferentiated, and residual. However, DSM-5 removed any mention of such types.

At times in the past, chronic, acute, and latent forms were also recognized. More recently, a distinction has been drawn between *deficit schizophrenia* and *non-deficit schizophrenia*, where the former syndrome denotes an especially heavy load of persistent negative symptoms (such as diminished affect, poverty of speech, and reduced motivation). Other investigators have examined whether there are discrete types of cognitive impairments. For example, some patients might suffer only from memory problems, while other patients might have problems in maintaining attentive states.[7] Whether any of the categorical distinctions mentioned in this paragraph are real or useful remains an open question.

People who have schizophrenia also differ significantly in respect to a range of biological measures. Many, but not all, patients with schizophrenia find it difficult to track moving targets with their eyes. Also, according to a Norwegian study, patients who have schizophrenia can be distinguished by how much polyunsaturated fatty acid they carry in their red blood cells.[8] Evidently, most patients have normal levels, but one-third of the patients have levels that are 80 percent lower. The difference is not accounted for by smoking habits, diet, medications, age, or gender but could be explained by one or more metabolic deficiencies in the low-level group. Other researchers have noted the highly variable responses of patients to antipsychotic medications.

Thus, like cancer, schizophrenia may comprise different but related disorders. Although all cancers are caused by the uncontrolled proliferation of cells, more than 100 different types of cancer can be distinguished on the basis of their locations in the body, the types of tissues that are affected, and whether they create hard tumor masses. Similarly, even though all cases of schizophrenia are likely caused by faulty brain development, some types may have abnormalities mostly in the prefrontal cortex, and other types may be centered in the hippocampus, or elsewhere. Nonfunctional glutamate receptors may be the root cause in some cases, while improper fiber connections may be the cause in other cases.

Now, recall that many different genes are implicated in causing both schizophrenia and cancer. In respect to cancer, different mutations underlie malignant growths in different types of tissues, and even breast cancer, which was once regarded as a single type, is now known to comprise at least ten subtypes on the basis of genetic profiles.[9] Schizophrenia, too, probably comprises subtypes distinguished by genetics. If, as many researchers believe, there are dozens or perhaps even thousands of mutations that contribute to the risk of schizophrenia, then clearly different combinations of risk genes could create different symptoms by acting on different parts of the brain.

As a further complication, there now appear to be good reasons for questioning Emil Kraepelin's historic division of mental illnesses into schizophrenia on one side and mood-affecting disorders on the other side. For starters, the symptoms of schizophrenia overlap with those of bipolar disorder. Psychosis occurs in both. The positive symptoms of schizophrenia (delusions, hallucinations, and disorganized speech) are common during the manic phase of bipolar disorder, and the negative symptoms of schizophrenia (low affect, social withdrawal, and apathy) are common in the depressive phase of bipolar disorder. The neurotransmitters serotonin and dopamine are implicated in both diseases, and several medications that were originally developed for one disease have subsequently been found effective for the other disease.

Nor is schizophrenia clearly distinct from autism. The hallmarks of autism, limited social interactions and bizarre behaviors, are so similar to symptoms in schizophrenia that autism was regarded as childhood schizophrenia up until the 1970s. Moreover, researchers in Scandinavia have uncovered family links between schizophrenia and autism.[10] After analyzing large Swedish databases, they found that children with autism were 2.9 times more likely to have a parent with schizophrenia than were healthy children, and the children with autism were 2.6 times more likely to have a sibling with schizophrenia. Similar results were obtained in Denmark. Autism was also associated with bipolar disease, but to a lesser extent. As noted earlier, data such as these suggest a genetic basis for the family associations, but they do not rule out environmental influences.

Compelling evidence for a genetic link between various psychiatric disorders comes from studies of risk factors. In early studies, several specific genes, including *ANK3*, *CACNA1C*, and *ZNF804A*, were found to be associated with both schizophrenia and bipolar disorder. More recently, an international team of researchers used powerful molecular and statistical methods to analyze the genomes of 33,332 patients and 27,888 mentally healthy persons. The group discovered four genetic variants that are significant risk factors for five disorders: schizophrenia, bipolar disorder, autism, major depression, and attention deficit-hyperactivity disorder.[11] The data parallel those from other studies in which certain gene variants were found to be risk factors for many different autoimmune disorders, including rheumatoid arthritis, multiple sclerosis, systemic lupus erythematosus, psoriasis, Crohn's disease, and type 1 diabetes. Together, the studies underscore the fact that some gene variants can cause a variety of different medical conditions within a single functional system.

The genetic evidence suggests an intriguing common mechanism for the five psychiatric disorders noted above, because two of the four variants identified in that study appear to affect the same brain structure. Both of them make a protein component of a channel in nerve cell membranes through which calcium flows. There are five types of calcium channels, but these two genetic variants build only the L type. Because the L type calcium channel has numerous important roles in both the construction of the adult brain and its subsequent functioning, it is possible that defects in the calcium channel cause brain alterations that lead to any one of several psychiatric illnesses, depending on other factors.

Problems with the concept of schizophrenia have led a growing number of experts to reject altogether the notion that schizophrenia is a distinct disease. At the beginning of this chapter, I quoted an article that said that the concept of schizophrenia is "mired in controversy and remains unsatisfactory." After reviewing the relevant facts, the authors went on to state, "This body of facts leads us to conclude that the current world of schizophrenia likely includes multiple . . . overlapping syndromes and diseases, and that the unitary concept of schizophrenia may have outlived its usefulness."[12] A different group of mental health researchers has made a similar appeal, asking us to think of schizophrenia as just one member in a group of "related and overlapping syndromes that result in part from a combination of genetic and environmental effects on brain development and that are associated with specific and general impairments of cognitive function."[13] Both sets of authors maintain that there are no consistent or unique features of schizophrenia that separate it from other mental conditions, especially those involving psychosis.

Instead of worrying about how to bundle the symptoms of mental illnesses into neat categories, investigators and clinicians alike are looking for alternative approaches. Many are beginning to think in terms of specific abnormalities that cut across diagnostic categories, abnormalities such as hallucinations, lack of affect, and depression. Some reformers even want to eliminate what they see as the unnecessary boundary between mental illness and normality. Nearly everyone has heard internal voices; most people are familiar with the feeling of paranoia; and it is not unusual, in times of stress, to withdraw from social situations. The reformers are attempting to unravel the causal relationships between specific gene variants, specific brain abnormalities, and specific behavioral or psychological symptoms.[14] This type of research, they say, will provide insights that can lead to effective treatments. One example of the approach is the focus on the prefrontal cortex, where genes and the environment are known to interact, and where progress has been made in understanding the cellular mechanisms that underlie the lobe's unique functions.

SUMMARY

- Emil Kraepelin gave the first full description of a newly recognized mental disease in 1893. He called it dementia praecox, but the name was changed to schizophrenia in 1911. Ever since, people have struggled to agree on a precise definition.
- Current diagnostic manuals rely on psychological and behavioral criteria that require subjective judgments. Doctors must make all-or-none decisions about the presence or absence of symptoms and adhere to rigid diagnostic rules. Although the use of biological tests could improve the reliability of diagnoses, no such test has yet been validated.
- Schizophrenia is a heterogeneous disease with symptoms that vary widely from patient to patient. Numerous subtypes have been proposed on the basis of psychological, biological, and other criteria. In

the future, genetic profiling will likely provide the most reliable basis for distinguishing schizophrenia subtypes.

- People with bipolar disorder can have hallucinations and delusions during the manic phase, and they feel apathetic during the depressive phase. Thus, the symptoms of bipolar disease overlap with the symptoms of schizophrenia. Also, the two diseases share certain genetic risk factors. These considerations suggest that bipolar disorder and schizophrenia may not be truly distinct. Similar examples of overlap exist between other categories of mental illness.

- A growing number of experts are abandoning the concept of schizophrenia as a single, well-defined disease. They are beginning to focus their research on specific symptoms of cognitive and behavioral dysfunction, with the objective of understanding the origins and mechanisms of each individual impairment.

- Even though schizophrenia may be nothing more than a convenient catchword for a range of mental disorders, we have little choice but to continue using the term until scientific research forces a new conceptualization.

17

Libraries and Literature

My brother's next stop was a board-and-care facility in Pasadena, located about a mile from the Rose Bowl, the stadium where all of us in the family, often together, had watched college football over the years. The name of the residence, Castle Hill, was yet another of Mrs. Nelson's euphemisms. It presumably referred to the fantasy structure on the adjacent property in which, ironically, I had partied many years earlier. Just as we had hoped, Jim's spirit lifted after his move to Castle Hill.

Jim had his own room, the grounds were more attractive than in the Centinela Retirement Home, and the nearby streets were more inviting for walks. He especially liked its proximity to a public library, because he felt at home in libraries. The only jobs he ever had (both of them part-time) were in libraries. As an undergraduate student at UCLA, he worked in the Powell Undergraduate Library and later, after hospitalization, he worked in the library of the Neuropsychiatric Institute and Hospital at UCLA. In Pasadena, he made frequent visits to the local library.

Once, when I asked Jim about the library, he replied that he had stopped going there. He explained that nonmembers were no longer permitted in the building, which was obviously a falsehood. More likely, I suspect, some of the library's patrons had noticed Jim and had become upset by his behavior or even by his mere presence. It must have been like what had happened at the Ambassador Hotel back when he was living at the Portland Villa. In any case, I said nothing further about it. As events unfolded, however, the library story marked the beginning of the end for Jim. His mental condition began to deteriorate and, three years later, as a result of the medication that he was taking, he experienced a medical emergency that ultimately led to his death. Before that happened, however, I had some good visits with Jim in Pasadena. One of the most memorable was also the last occasion Jim and his father spent time together.

Pasadena lies at the eastern edge of the Los Angeles basin and thus far from Westwood Village and the usual destinations of the Chase family. Nevertheless, we had special attachments to the city. It was, after all, our first stop in California after trekking from Chicago. Also, we loved the romance of the giant parade that filled the streets of central Pasadena every New Year's Day. More than once, we left Westwood early in the morning on the first of January to join the hundreds of thousands of people lining the streets to see it; in all other years we watched the parade on TV. And, if we were not in the stadium for the celebrated Rose Bowl football game, we would watch it too on TV. Our more serious devotion, however, was reserved for the Huntington Library, an institution renowned for its historical collection of significant books, its magnificent gardens, and its splendid art gallery. And so, it was to be expected that when Dad came with me to see Jim in Pasadena, the three of us would travel the short distance to San Marino and the Huntington Library. Jim's previous visit to the library had been in 1948, the year of our arrival in California.

"Jim," I asked, "What would you like to see first, the books or the gardens?" As if I didn't know.

We proceeded to the rare books collection, where every display case in every room holds a literary masterpiece or a historical gem. There is a copy of the so-called Gutenberg Bible from 1450, the first book printed with movable type; a first folio edition of Shakespeare's collected plays, dated 1623; and a lavishly illustrated manuscript copy of Chaucer's *Canterbury Tales*, thought to have been produced around 1410. More than any other item, however, it was the 1726 edition of Jonathan Swift's *Gulliver's Travels* that drew Jim's sustained attention. He peered silently over the display case for what seemed a very long time. Finally, I felt compelled to nudge him along. Dad's favorite items were the handwritten letters of Abraham Lincoln, while my favorite was the gigantic

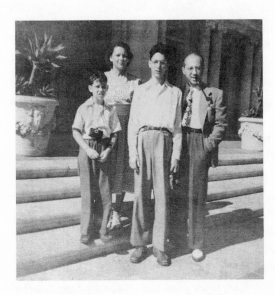

The Chase family at the
Huntington Library in
San Marino, 1948

first-edition copy of John James Audubon's *Birds of America*. Curiously, as we moved from display to display, Jim spoke hardly at all. I imagine that he was stupefied by these tangible encounters with his literary heroes.

After the books, as we walked to the gallery of paintings, we spoke excitedly about revisiting Thomas Gainsborough's magnificent *Blue Boy* and his companion *Pinkie* by Thomas Lawrence. These beautiful portraits did not disappoint us. Afterward, we headed back toward the entrance, but by now we had traveled a considerable distance, and the way back required us to walk the length of the horticultural garden. Dad, who was 95 years old, was having a hard time of it. I offered to get him a wheelchair, but he insisted on walking, so we proceeded very slowly and with frequent rests. I suffered in sympathy with my father's pain, and I suppose Jim did too. When we eventually arrived at the reception area, I suggested that we stop in the café to rest.

Jim wolfed down a generous portion of his favorite dish, pancakes with butter and syrup; Dad had hot soup and a salad, and I had a tuna fish sandwich. The food and drink revived us, and as we sat there, the talk turned to literature and authors.

I began by remarking that I was disappointed that there were no works of Aldous Huxley in the library. "I suppose he's too recent for this place," I said. "What do you think, Jim? He's one of your favorites, isn't he?"

"*Antic Hay* is a fine book. So too is *Crome Yellow*. It's his first novel, if I'm not mistaken. These books show that Huxley was a precocious intellect. He was to become one of the most important writers of his generation."

"I never read those books. *Brave New World* and *Island*—those are my favorites."

"Yes," Jim said, "and then there are his essays. Actually, most of his novels read like essays, but they are masterfully written."

I then broached a subject that had long intrigued me. Could Jim's interest in Huxley have anything to do with the latter's experiments with hallucinogenic drugs? I was pretty sure that Jim had experienced hallucinations, so I asked him, "What about *The Doors of Perception*? What did you think of it?" This book, the title of which is taken from a poem by William Blake, tells of a single, eight-hour experiment with the hallucinogenic drug mescaline. My curiosity to know Jim's take on Huxley's much praised account of that day was abruptly squashed when Jim declared that he had never read the book. So much for that speculation.

I continued trying to draw out my brother on subjects that were close to his interests; I wanted to hear him express himself with more feeling. Thus, when Jim remarked that he enjoyed seeing the first folio edition of Shakespeare's plays, I asked him if he had a favorite play. He replied that he was more familiar with Shakespeare's sonnets, so again I queried his favorite.

"*When in disgrace with fortune* is considered one of his finest." And then, astonishingly, Jim recited the entire sonnet with hardly a pause.

When, in disgrace with fortune and men's eyes,
I all alone beweep my outcast state
And trouble deaf heaven with my bootless cries
And look upon myself and curse my fate,
Wishing me like to one more rich in hope,

Featured like him, like him with friends possess'd,
Desiring this man's art and that man's scope,
With what I most enjoy contented least;
Yet in these thoughts myself almost despising,
Haply I think on thee, and then my state,
Like to the lark at break of day arising
From sullen earth, sings hymns at heaven's gate;
For thy sweet love remember'd such wealth brings
That then I scorn to change my state with kings.

Dad and I sat back in stunned amazement. What a performance! Contrary to some of the statements that I have read in the psychiatric literature about people with schizophrenia suffering from poor memories, Jim had an excellent memory. Jim even had a good autobiographical memory, the memory of personal experiences, which the psychiatrists say is especially impaired in schizophrenia. Jim remembered many family events that I had forgotten. As I have said, the symptoms of schizophrenia vary widely among individuals.

Having had the opportunity to rest, Dad was also feeling better now. He too liked to encourage Jim's interest in literature, so he trotted out some names to elicit Jim's comments: T. S. Eliot, Christopher Isherwood (an acquaintance of Jim's from UCLA), James Joyce, and *his* favorite poet, Edgar Allan Poe. Before long, Dad was also reciting,

It was many and many a year ago,
In a kingdom by the sea,
That a maiden there lived whom you may know
By the name of Annabel Lee;
And this maiden she lived with no other thought
Than to love and be loved by me.

He went on for another two stanzas, but he was unable to complete all six, as was always the case with Dad's recitations of this poem.

Dad asked Jim about some other Poe poems, but Jim coldly ignored him.

Jim had a difficult, ambivalent relationship with Dad. Having finally accepted Jim's illness, Dad was invariably gentle with him, and he supported him in every way that he could, but the warmth was not always reciprocated. At times, Jim seemed in awe of Dad, while at other times he seemed to fear him. I was never able to figure out what, exactly, was at the root of their strained relationship. In any case, Jim's conversations with Dad were often hesitant, awkward affairs, and it fell upon me to mediate their relationship. It did not surprise me, therefore, when Jim ignored Dad's invitation to extend the discussion about literature.

As we got up to leave, Jim announced that he wanted to buy some pastries for a woman friend at Castle Hill. I didn't know if he could manage the transaction, so I offered to get the pastries for him. But he said, no, he would do it himself. Sure enough, he went to the counter, purchased two chocolate croissants, and proudly carried the small bag to our car. A trivial event, one might say, but like Jim's purchase of shoes in Inglewood, it stuck in my mind. I remember these events because they epitomize how far removed from the ordinary world of commercial transactions Jim's life in the board-and-care homes had become. Or perhaps they only show that I had a low estimation of his social skills. Regardless, Jim's thoughtful gesture on behalf of his friend touched me.

Jim's education had prepared him for a career as either a professor of English literature or creative author. He entertained both ambitions until his illness took hold, after which all of that went by the wayside. Nevertheless, he left a literary legacy, albeit one considerably smaller than any represented at the Huntington Library. Most of his writing was in the form of letters addressed to me. In addition, he occasionally kept a journal, and he wrote a few poems and some short pieces of nonfiction. None of his works from before his illness remain, and of his later works, I regret to say that only a portion remains. Nevertheless, there are documents that, when read, bring to life the echo of Jim's voice.

Jim's most creative period coincided with the years immediately after his first psychotic crisis, when he was between the ages of 25 and 27. At this time, he viewed himself—rightly so—as an intellectual author with something to say. Apart from the letters, the longest of his works consist of just a few typewritten pages, and they are mostly about women: Sally, who sat next to him in a graduate course on Elizabethan poetry before she killed herself; Charlotte, a classmate from high school who crossed paths with Jim in the hospital; and an unnamed blonde girl whom Jim had tried to pick up at a bus stop (story entitled *The Night on Fire*). In one thoughtful piece, Jim describes Dad's personality; in another he gives a short account of Mom driving him to see Dr. Held. He wrote a few epigrams on diverse subjects (*Wilshire Boulevard*, *Rain*, *My Lamp*).

Here is the unedited beginning of his little story about Joan, a patient at his hospital whom he had dared to kiss:

> I woke up one morning in the hospital and heard a girl talking loudly and continuously in the hall; my senses quickened with sexual appetite: a woman, a female, was there, in my imagination to be taken. I put on my robe, threw a towel over my shoulder, and went out into the hall. She came over to me and looked up at me directly; she was half a foot shorter than I; she had on her pajamas, no make-up, and her hair was disheveled; a ceremonious meeting.
>
> "Hi. What do you do?"
>
> "I don't do anything. I'm a bum."
>
> She scowled.
>
> "Come on now, what do you *do*? What's your name? My name's Joan. I'm married and I've got a kid. What's your name?"
>
> "My name is René Descartes, and I have ten kids."

Later in the story:

> I was flattered [by her attentions] even if the first woman to care for me (aside from my mother) was a sick woman. I thought about sickness and health. It seemed to me that the people in the hospital were more sensitive, more finely put together, than their counterparts on the outside; the easy conclusion was that their illness and their finer qualities were necessary to each other, causes of each other, and that to cure their illness would be to destroy their finer qualities. But I could not believe that. Anyone could become ill: therefore anyone could be well. Some types of people were more easily derailed than others; it was like a butcher's scale and a chemist's scale, the one was more delicate, more easily unbalanced than the other.

And superior qualities, I decided, existed not because of, but in spite of neurosis; they were two frogs sitting side by side, uncommunicative.

And the climax:

> Let us be precise about these matters. We kissed many many times; Joan counted them. She was the first woman I had kissed since my mother. We had to wait until no attendants were looking, and when we were finished I quickly wiped the lipstick off my lips. (She had put make-up on, and looked very feminine.) I covered three handkerchiefs with her rosy tint. We walked arm in arm up and down the hall, about 15 yards, and pretended it was the Champs-Elysée, and the ladder standing at one end the Tour Eiffel.

In contrast to the narrative pieces and essays, which were rather forced and self-conscious, Jim's letters were free and reflective of his moods. When I was at university (in the early years of his illness), he and I exchanged letters nearly every week. Later, after I moved to the East Coast of the United States, and then to Canada, his letters continued to arrive, but less often. All together, I received several hundred letters from my brother. The early letters were filled with commentaries on literature, political opinions, and sporting news (mostly baseball and football). He occasionally offered his philosophical reflections on life and from time to time attempted to analyze his psychological condition.

As the years wore on, the letters increasingly centered on his struggles and his regrets. The quality of his writing declined, and the frequently fragmented sentences became less than lucid and occasionally plainly irrational. Nevertheless, his intelligence and his use of irony— whether intentional or not—remained intact. Here are some verbatim excerpts from his final letter to me, dated October 24, 1994.

> How goes it? Here, I am in such a idiotic place that I want *out*—O.U.T. My frustration is extreme. I am a fish-out-of-water, with no-one to talk to, nor even a television set to watch. I remain a poor, premier, sorely beset example of the schizo. type. It is a Kafka-esque situation.
>
> I may not be "premier," but the schizo. illness does take a toll. For me, it was the disparity between (Ah, between) body and mind. Terrible difficulty in human relations. Lack of an occupation.

I read too many books, but did not grasp them very well. People, as you, tell me that I am *cut out* to work in a library. I agree. Clean, quiet, detailed work and doing a service. Library Assistant. Donne's poetry, you know, was not published in his lifetime. [Here Jim may be responding to my mention of Donne in an earlier letter.] It was widely circulated in manuscript. The great, sensual metaphor the wit and the truth of the love expressed, are superb. "And therefore never send to know for whom the bell tolls . . ." Hemingway's title, as you know.

When Did Schizophrenia First Appear, and Why Doesn't It Go Away?

When I became a professional biologist, I was told, "Nothing in biology makes sense except in the light of evolution."[1] I began to think about the evolution of schizophrenia. Once I realized that there is a physical basis to the disease, that it is not caused solely by environmental factors, and that genes play a major role in determining who gets it, I recognized a fundamental evolutionary paradox. If schizophrenia is so obviously bad for those who have it, why have the mutations that make people vulnerable to schizophrenia persisted through human history? To better understand this paradox, we need to begin by reviewing the basic principles of evolution.

Charles Darwin wrote that evolution occurs only when individual traits vary within a species, as when a particular bone is longer in some individuals than in others. Some variations may, for whatever reason, cause the individuals who possess them to produce more offspring. If so, and provided that the variations are heritable, these variations will tend to become more common in the population; this is called *positive selection*. Other variations will, somehow, cause the individuals who possess them to produce fewer offspring, and these variations will tend to become less common in the population; this is called *negative selection*. Because we now know (although Darwin did not) that traits are inherited through the bits of deoxyribonucleic acid which constitute genes, we can say that it is the variation in *genes* that is the true basis of evolution.

Schizophrenia is a trait whose presence varies throughout the population. Thus, even though schizophrenia makes people unhappy, socially dysfunctional, and cognitively impaired, the only thing that matters for the evolution of schizophrenia is whether affects an individual's ability to pass along his or her genes to the next generation, that is, to reproduce.[2] Here the facts are quite clear. Fourteen independent studies compared the fertility rates (number of offspring per individual) for people with schizophrenia and for healthy individuals who were matched with them on the basis of age, gender, and other demographic variables.[3] In all but one of these studies, the fertility of the schizophrenia group was well below that of the non-schizophrenia group.

By far the largest and best controlled of these studies was conducted in Finland using a public registry of 11,231 schizophrenia patients. In this study, the fertility of female schizophrenia patients was 45 percent of the fertility for females in the general population, and the fertility of the male patients was just 27 percent of the fertility for males in the general population. An analysis of these data indicated that the low fertility rates were due to the inability of the people with schizophrenia to attract and retain mates, not because they died prematurely. Regardless, there can be no doubt that people with schizophrenia leave few offspring, and that fact forms the basis of an evolutionary paradox. Why has negative selection not caused schizophrenia to disappear? Before I attempt to answer this question, and to resolve the paradox, I pause to explain a key difference between evolutionary biology and most other areas of biology.

While all of biology, like science in general, is concerned with causes, evolutionary biology is unique because it relies very little on experiments and measurements. Its methods *must* be different, because the causes that it seeks to discover occurred in the long ago past. So, to understand what caused a trait to evolve or to explain why it persists, evolutionary biologists use a combination of present-day observations and basic principles to draw inferences about past events. Those principles originated with Charles Darwin in the mid-nineteenth century, but they have been subsequently elaborated and modified. Even today, there remains room for the development of evolutionary theory, and when it comes to explaining the evolutionary history of particular traits, outright speculation is not uncommon. Not surprisingly, therefore, those scientists who seek to explain the evolutionary paradox of schizophrenia often debate one another in the scholarly literature. I will summarize the substance of their arguments in the remainder of this chapter.[4]

One approach to the evolutionary paradox of schizophrenia is to say, okay, people living today with schizophrenia may leave few offspring, but what about in earlier times. Perhaps schizophrenia was not such a bad thing long ago. The genes that cause schizophrenia might have been less damaging in the prehistoric era if the symptoms had been milder or if people had been more tolerant of affected individuals. Indeed, if people with schizophrenia were seen as gifted shamans, they might even have been favored as mating partners. According to these scenarios, the risk genes became harmful so recently that selection has not yet had time to weed them out.

Opponents of this argument point out that it is incompatible with the rate at which negative selection is known to eliminate disadvantageous genes. Two researchers did a simple calculation. They took as their starting point the assumption that schizophrenia has been harmful to fertility only since the year 1600.[5] That is, they assumed that negative selection against the causative genes has been operating for only about 20 generations. They then used the current prevalence of schizophrenia in Finland and the rate of gene elimination by negative selection to estimate that 42 percent of Finns must have had schizophrenia in 1600. Because this is an absurd inference, these authors reject the notion that schizophrenia survives today because it has only recently become harmful.[6]

Alternatively, schizophrenia might persist because the genetic mutations that reduce fertility through schizophrenia have additional effects that actually *increase* fertility. If, as a result, the net effect on fertility is minimal or even slightly positive, the mutations will remain prevalent. This explanation, known as *balancing selection*, is popular with both evolutionary biologists and the public. It could work in any one of several ways. One possibility is based on the example of sickle-cell anemia. Every person carries two copies (two **alleles**) of each gene. In sickle-cell anemia, there exist two alleles of a gene that encodes a blood protein; we can refer to these variants as *a* and *A*. If someone has two copies of the *a* allele (*aa*), he or she is at risk for sickle-cell anemia.

On the other hand, if someone has two copies of the *A* allele (*AA*), he or she is susceptible to malaria. As for the third possibility, one copy of the *a* allele and one copy of the *A* allele (*Aa*), people with this genotype are resistant to both sickle-cell anemia and malaria. Thus, while both sickle-cell anemia and malaria have harmful effects that reduce fertility, neither variant has been eliminated from our genome because the *combination* of the two variants is beneficial; each variant is required to prevent double copies of the other variant. Good and bad consequences of a genetic mutation can balance each other and create conditions to block negative selection. Something like this could be happening with schizophrenia.

Another version of balancing selection imagines that a single allele has two different effects. The hypothesis assumes that while negative selection acts to eliminate a mutation that causes schizophrenia and thereby *reduces* fertility, positive selection acts simultaneously to preserve the same mutation because it *enhances* fertility through some other trait. The scenario envisions a trade-off between good and bad effects, as the result of which the disease-causing mutation persists.

An unlikely quartet of authors first applied this version of balancing selection theory to schizophrenia in 1964. One author was Julian Huxley, the biologist brother of the celebrated author Aldous Huxley, and the first head of the United Nations Education, Cultural and Scientific Organization (UNESCO); another author was Ernst Mayr, the distinguished professor of evolutionary zoology at Harvard University; the remaining authors were Humphry Osmond, a British psychiatrist who used the psychedelic drug LSD in therapies, and Abram Hoffer, a Canadian psychiatrist who prescribed megavitamins for schizophrenia. Writing in the international journal of science, *Nature*, these authors proposed that the genes that create the risk of schizophrenia also deliver "physiological advantages," suggesting that they might protect against such things as bodily wounds, high levels of circulating insulin, allergies, and infections. Although the article's four authors presented no evidence for any of these particular advantages—all seem highly unlikely—other respected authors have championed different traits as possible trade-offs for schizophrenia. Let us examine the cases for and against the most plausible of these hypotheses.

Some people believe that the risk of schizophrenia is balanced by high intelligence. The idea gained popularity after the release of the book and movie *A Beautiful Mind*, celebrating the life of John Forbes Nash, the Nobel Prize–winning mathematician. He was a remarkable individual, but his example alone does not prove the hypothesis. My brother was also very intelligent, and he told me about a patient in one of the psychiatric hospitals who was reputed to have an IQ of 165, which would have placed him in the "genius" category. This fellow played chess with Jim, but he never won a single game, and he took forever to make his moves; he thought that all white pieces were virtuous and all black pieces were evil. There are no doubt other very smart people with schizophrenia, proving only that anyone can get the disease. To determine the true relationship between intelligence, measured by IQ tests, and the risk of schizophrenia, one needs to obtain IQ scores from people before any of them get schizophrenia (a prospective study). The results show that the IQs of people who later develop schizophrenia are, on average, *lower*, not higher, than the IQs of people who remain mentally healthy. Moreover, the *lower* the IQ score, the greater is the risk of schizophrenia. Clearly, the genes that confer the risk of schizophrenia do not also provide the advantage of high intelligence.

Another hypothesis proposes that schizophrenia emerged very early in human evolution in conjunction with certain crucial traits.[7] In this scenario, schizophrenia is the by-product or necessary companion of these species-defining traits. Most of the speculation concerns language and complex social arrangements, both of which are thought to have evolved shortly before *Homo sapiens* migrated out of Africa, about 70,000 years ago. Language and social adaptations were made possible by genetic mutations that changed the structure of the brain. Some theorists believe that these changes made the brain vulnerable to schizophrenia. Even though schizophrenia was maladaptive, it could not be eliminated by negative selection because the genes that caused it were needed to sustain human evolution.

So goes the argument, but there are factual and theoretical problems. Mainly, if schizophrenia risk genes appeared so early in human history, and if they are linked to language and social organization, which are universal human traits, one would expect that the genes would be uniformly distributed and that all people would have an equal risk of schizophrenia. However, epidemiological research does not bear out this prediction; on the contrary, the incidence of schizophrenia varies considerably among different groups of people and in different regions of the world.[8]

While each of the preceding versions of the balancing selection hypothesis has its backers, the most popular by far focuses on human creativity as the benefit that balances the risk of schizophrenia. Advocates of this hypothesis see signs of creativity in the hallucinations, delusions, and bizarre behaviors of people with schizophrenia. This hypothesis, like the one about high intelligence, has drawn support from the example of John Forbes Nash, who has schizophrenia but is also highly creative. He, however, is exceptional. Moreover, it is inappropriate to lump together as "creative" Nash's mathematical genius and his hallucinations. In reality, hallucinations and delusions, the two cardinal symptoms of psychosis, are not really creative because they are involuntary and maladaptive. Research shows that, once psychotic symptoms are put aside, people with schizophrenia are no more creative than people who live free of the disease. And, anyway, even if they were more creative, they are still less fertile.

Despite these objections, advocates of the creativity hypothesis point to evidence suggesting that the close relatives of people with schizophrenia or related mental disorders may be somewhat more creative than average.[9] Furthermore, researchers have found that certain cognitive styles relating to "divergent thinking" can be observed in poets and visual artists, as well as in people who have schizophrenia. One way to interpret these findings is to suppose that individuals who have low or moderate doses of certain genes are exceptionally creative, whereas individuals with high doses of the same genes get schizophrenia. Possibly, the symptoms of schizophrenia suppress or hide that which would otherwise appear as exceptional creativity. The idea could be tested by conducting a prospective study in which creativity is measured in a large group of young people before any of them get schizophrenia, as in the IQ studies mentioned above. The creativity hypothesis predicts that the individuals who later develop schizophrenia would already show signs of exceptional creativity in their youth. Regrettably, no such study has yet been undertaken.

Ultimately, for creativity to work as an explanation for the persistence of schizophrenia, it must be shown that the benefits of high creativity include enhanced fertility. Somehow, the increased fertility from creativity must balance the reduced fertility from schizophrenia. Some support for this prediction comes from a British study that found that poets and artists had more sexual partners than did a random selection of adults who were matched on age, sex, and social class.[10] The next question is whether the healthy relatives of people with schizophrenia, who may be unusually creative, have increased numbers of sexual partners or increased numbers of children. Disappointingly, the preponderance of evidence finds no enhanced fertility for the relatives of people with schizophrenia.[11] This finding is highly damaging not only to the creativity hypothesis but also to all other versions of the balancing selection hypothesis, because it shows that the relatives do not have *any* fertility-enhancing traits associated with schizophrenia.

Considering all the evidence currently available, the idea that there is an evolutionary benefit associated with schizophrenia can probably be dismissed as unfounded speculation. Critics point out that people with Down syndrome have high self-esteem and are said to be cheerful and helpful. As well, psychological depression saves energy in the winter, mania boosts energy in the spring, and patients who are unable to feel pain enjoy a certain freedom. But these so-called benefits do not prevent persons with these illnesses from having low fertility rates. Citing the lack of evidence for reproductive benefits, and noting other objections such as those mentioned above, one prominent researcher dismisses all theories of balancing selection for schizophrenia, calling them "romantic and quasi-heroic." Dr. John McGrath believes that they arise from social and moral concerns rather than scientific facts.[12]

Fortunately, there are other types of evolutionary arguments. One particularly attractive idea is based on the fact that the evolution of traits entails two sources of selection, as described by Charles Darwin. Traits that are selected by the environment, broadly defined, come under the term *natural selection*. Thus, traits that help animals (or humans) to reproduce in certain climates, with certain food resources, or despite the presence of certain predators become fixed in the population through positive selection, whereas traits whose interactions with the environment lead to few or no offspring disappear through negative selection.

In addition, Darwin pointed out, some traits are selected (both positively and negatively) through a process that Darwin called *sexual selection*. Sexual selection operates when we choose our mates, but also when we compete with other individuals of the same sex for a mate whom we both want. The male peacock's tail is an example of a trait that was selected because it attracts females, and the ram's horns were selected because they give an edge in male-on-male competitions. In humans, height and breast size are two traits whose evolution has been influenced by sexual selection. A team of psychiatrists and evolutionary psychologists, led by Dr. Andrew Shaner at UCLA, has proposed that schizophrenia is the unfortunate consequence of a sexually selected trait.[13]

Dr. Shaner and his colleagues do not know what, exactly, is the sexually selected trait that is associated with schizophrenia, but they believe that it is something that helps a person attract mates. It could be creativity in the broad sense or, as the authors suggest, it could be something more specific, such as "verbal courtship behavior (e.g., attracting mates by telling funny stories . . . , social sensitivity, and emotional expressiveness)." Now, the male peacock's large and colorful tail attracts hens not because the tail is valuable in itself but because it indicates, or signals, that its bearer is an individual of high genetic quality. That is, any male bird that can display such a magnificent tail will be able to provide the hen with strong, healthy offspring. Why, then, do some male peacocks have ugly tails? The answer is, because they cannot help it; if they do not have the right genes, they will not have a beautiful tail. The ugly tail indicates that *its* bearer is a bird of *inferior* quality, a cock that the hen would be better off *not* mating with.

According to the hypothesis that I am presenting, schizophrenia in humans is like the male peacock's unattractive tail, except that it operates in both males and females. The symptoms of schizophrenia signal to potential mates that the afflicted individual is poorly qualified to become a partner in parenthood. In this view, the gene mutations that lead to impaired brain function also degrade one indicator of reproductive potential, namely, the engaging sexual personality. Dr. Shaner and his colleagues conclude, "Schizophrenia itself is not adaptive. Rather, it is the unattractive and dysfunctional . . . extreme of a highly variable trait that evolved for courtship." Evolution may have given us schizophrenia as the necessary counterpart to successful courtship.

A final scenario offers a relatively simple, and highly plausible, explanation for the persistence of schizophrenia. It is built on the fact that about 12,000 genes (approximately one-half of all human genes) make proteins exclusively in the brain. Even though genes rarely mutate spontaneously, because so many are at play in the brain there is a reasonable chance that, from time to time, at least one of these genes will be altered by a mutation. A recent analysis concluded that, on average, about one new harmful mutation appears in each newborn child, meaning that, on average, one of every two children has a new mutation in a brain-related gene.[14] In total, owing to the accumulation of mutations through successive generations, each human brain is thought to be affected by more than 500 mutations. While most of the mutations can be expected to have only insignificant effects, others can disrupt anything from neuronal chemistry to large-scale neural circuitry. Because the various parts of the brain are so interconnected and the brain's mechanisms so complex, even a single mutation can affect several neural processes with potentially serious consequences for cognition and behavior. And, because normal brain function can be disrupted in so many different ways, each mutation is likely to create a different set of symptoms, which fits nicely with the suggestion, mentioned earlier, that schizophrenia is a disease of heterogeneous symptoms, or even that it is a group of related, but genetically distinct, disorders.

Harmful mutations are ordinarily subject to negative selection, but in the time taken to eliminate one mutation in one gene, a new mutation is likely to appear in another gene. So long as the rate of mutation keeps up with the rate of elimination, there will always be mutations present in the human population that are capable of disrupting brain function and hence capable of producing schizophrenia. Moreover, as recent investigations have shown,[15] the number of mutations in the human genome has increased enormously in the past few millennia owing to the rapid expansion of the worldwide population. The mutations are appearing faster than they can be eliminated through negative selection.

Why has schizophrenia persisted is one question. Another question is this: *for how long* has it persisted? When, in fact, did schizophrenia begin? Although the whole of human evolution spans approximately 200,000 years, it would be difficult to verify the existence of schizophrenia before the appearance of literary texts, less than 5,000 years ago. But even written history contains few, if any, clearly recognizable descriptions of schizophrenia before the nineteenth century. Yes, there are passages in Hippocrates' writings and in early Greek dramas (*Orestes, Bacchae*) that refer to states of mental imbalance, and varieties of "madness" are depicted in Shakespeare's play *King Lear* (1608), especially in Lear himself and in Poor Tom, but do any of these examples constitute true schizophrenia? The fragmentary portrayals hardly allow a definitive diagnosis. According to the British psychiatrist Dr. Edward Hare, not a single unambiguous case of a patient hearing voices, that is, having an auditory hallucination, was recorded before the nineteenth century.[16] Given that auditory hallucinations are a hallmark of modern schizophrenia, the absence of such records suggests the absence of the disorder. It is not until the beginning of the nineteenth century that one finds credible descriptions of what we now call schizophrenia.

James Tilly Matthews was a tea broker in London when, from the gallery of the House of Commons, he shouted out that the home secretary was a traitor. Following his outburst, Matthews was admitted to the Bethlem psychiatric hospital in January 1797. There, he experienced conspiratorial fantasies and vivid hallucinations. The attending physician, John Haslam, wrote an entire book about Matthews, including a detailed description of the "air loom" machine, which, according to Matthews, emitted rays capable of tormenting Matthews and his political allies.[17] Haslam's account is the first comprehensive description of the disease that we now recognize as paranoid schizophrenia. From his knowledge of Matthews and other similar patients, Haslam announced a new type of "dementia" in the second edition of his psychiatric textbook, published in 1809. Independently, Philippe Pinel in France described the same disorder in the second edition of *his* textbook published in the same year. These initial descriptions of schizophrenia preceded Emil Kraepelin's elaboration of diagnostic criteria by about a hundred years.

Thus, it is tempting to speculate that schizophrenia first appeared around the year 1800. In any case, historians have noted that "the incidence of schizophrenia rose significantly during the 19th century."[18] The incidences of other mental disorders also increased at this time, and there was a dramatic increase in the total number of psychiatric patients residing in European asylums. Several factors were at play, including the greater recognition of psychiatric cases, problems with alcoholism and syphilis, and the longer duration of patients in the asylums. To determine how much of the overall increase in mental illness could be assigned to an increase in schizophrenia, Edward Hare poured though old hospital and government records. His striking conclusion is that "at least 40 percent of the increased prevalence of insanity between 1849 and 1909" can be attributed to an increase in the incidence of schizophrenia.[19]

We are left to ponder various scenarios. Possibly, schizophrenia emerged as a new disease at the beginning of the nineteenth century. Alternatively, it existed previously, but was extremely rare until the early part of the nineteenth century, at which time it became significantly more prevalent. According to an intermediate scenario, a preexisting disorder quickly changed from being relatively mild and relatively rare to become more severe and more common. Such a transformation might have come about as a consequence of new environmental toxins, new infectious agents, or new diets. Or a new mutation may have occurred in one or more genes.

SUMMARY

- From the perspective of evolutionary biology, the presence of schizophrenia in human populations is paradoxical. Because people with schizophrenia leave fewer offspring than do healthy individuals, theory predicts that the gene mutations that confer risk for the illness should be eliminated by negative selection.

- A popular hypothesis assumes a balancing scenario whereby the risk-causing genes persist because they bring beneficial effects along with the potentially harmful ones. Some scientists speculate that the risk of schizophrenia arose from mutations that changed our brains so that we could communicate using language. Others think that the harmful consequences of schizophrenia are balanced by high creativity.

- According to a different hypothesis, schizophrenia represents the negative extreme of a trait that is positively represented by skills in courtship. Schizophrenia may signal to potential sexual partners that the person carries mutated genes that will affect brain development and cause cognitive impairments. If so, schizophrenia may persist because it maintains the efficiency of mate selection.

- Even though harmful genes, such as those for schizophrenia, are eventually eliminated by negative selection, there are always new mutations. So long as the rate of new mutations exceeds the rate of elimination, the number of mutations in the human genome will continue to grow.

- Approximately 12,000 genes are active exclusively in the brain. Because normal brain functions depend upon a high degree of neural connectivity and a multitude of biochemical interactions, a single mutation in any one of these genes can disrupt normal brain activity, each in a different way. These facts may account for the diversity of schizophrenia symptoms.

- Potentially complicating all evolutionary scenarios is evidence suggesting either that schizophrenia first arose in the nineteenth century or that an older, related illness became much more severe at this time.

19

Jim's Final Days

It was mid-July, and all day hot air had been blowing into Pasadena from the desert. An hour earlier the manager at Castle Hill had phoned me to say that Jim had not yet returned from his customary walk. She was clearly worried, and so was I. When she phoned again a short while later to report that Jim had shown up, I was initially relieved, but then I worried anew when she added that he was dehydrated, confused, and refusing to eat or drink. A few days later, I flew to L.A., rented a car, and drove immediately to the Huntington Memorial Hospital in Pasadena where I found Jim in the respiratory unit. He was languishing in bed, looking awful, and saying little.

His doctor—young, but already arrogant—told me that Jim had a respiratory infection and that he was being treated with antibiotics. This seemed an odd diagnosis in light of what the Castle Hill manager had told me earlier. Stranger still was the fact that Jim, an indigent person, was occupying a large private room in this magnificent hospital. Perhaps there were no multipatient rooms at the hospital, or none available, but I doubt it. More likely, the medical staff wished to avoid problems with their unusual patient. I believe they put him in a private room to prevent him from disturbing other patients with his irrational behavior. When I later reflected on these circumstances, I came to realize that the staff's fear of trouble probably contributed to the more serious medical condition that ultimately killed Jim. More about this below.

Jim's condition gradually improved, but after 10 or so days in the Huntington Memorial Hospital, he was still not in good enough shape to return to Castle Hill. As his doctors and social workers deliberated about what to do with him, I tried but failed to have him transferred to an affiliated special unit for psychiatric medical patients. Instead, he was sent to the Centinela Valley Hospital, which is located in Inglewood immediately adjacent to the Centinela Retirement Home, where Jim had previously resided. From glimpses of the hospital that I recalled from my earlier visits to the home, I knew that the hospital was a very different kind of facility from the modern, immaculate Huntington Memorial Hospital. By this time I was already back in Montreal, but I did not like the fact that my brother was being cared for in such a miserable place, and my extreme unease was deepened by the difficulty I was having obtaining information about his condition. As it happened, his condition got worse, not better, and two weeks after arriving at the Centinela Valley Hospital, he was sent to the Los Angeles Metropolitan Hospital.

Once again, I quickly left for L.A. When I got there, I found Jim in an intensive care unit, curled up in a fetal position, unable to communicate, and looking just awful. From what I could see, and from scraps of information pulled from hospital staff, it seemed that all his body systems were failing. I was given to believe that he had only days to live. To make matters worse, the senior doctor who had first looked after him was on vacation, leaving a young gastro specialist in charge. Jim's fate now hung on the decisions of a man who was poorly prepared to deal with this type of case. I decided to share with him what I had learned in the medical library at McGill University in the days preceding my flight to L.A.

My wife, a nurse, had suggested to me that Jim's sudden physical deterioration might have been caused by his medications. Anxious for answers, I immersed myself in the psychiatric literature, where I read about a rare condition known as neuroleptic malignant syndrome (NMS), described as "an idiosyncratic, life-threatening complication of treatment with antipsychotic drugs that is characterized by fever, severe muscle rigidity, and autonomic and mental status changes." The word *neuroleptic* refers to antipsychotic medications. The exact causes of NMS are variable, but "nearly all case [studies] of NMS patients have reported physical exhaustion and dehydration prior to the onset of

NMS. Elevated environmental temperature has been proposed as a contributing factor in some [studies]."[1]

Because the description fit the facts in Jim's case, I considered that Jim may have already been suffering from NMS when he was admitted to the hospital in Pasadena. I recalled that he had spoken gibberish and referred to paranoid fantasies during a recent telephone conversation. Also, his caretakers had told me that Jim had become involved in fights. Once he ran naked into the common room and urinated on the carpet; another time, he threw a drinking glass full of water at a resident. Knowing that excessive antipsychotic medication can precipitate NMS, I guessed that the NMS could have started when the staff at Castle Hill increased his medications to combat his deteriorating mental state. Alternatively, maybe the NMS began only after he left Castle Hill. Maybe he did have a respiratory infection. In this scenario, the doctors' fear of incidents could have turned the infection into something far more serious when they administered antipsychotic drugs. They could have precipitated NMS by using a different drug from the one he had been accustomed to, increasing its dosage, or injecting it rather than administering it in pill form.

I wanted to speak to Jim's doctor because I knew that few physicians, even few psychiatrists, had heard of NMS in 1998. Before I was able to contact him, however, I visited Jim again in his hospital room. He lay rigid beneath his bed sheets, unable or unwilling to speak. A nurse informed me that because he was not eating, a tube had been inserted directly into his stomach so that he could be fed. Later that day the doctor phoned me, and I brazenly spilled out my newly acquired knowledge. Fortunately, the doctor listened carefully to what I had to say, and afterward he began administering Dantrolene, a drug that mimics the actions of dopamine and therefore reverses the pharmacological effects of antipsychotic (neuroleptic) medications. Two days later, the doctor phoned me to say that Jim's condition had improved "dramatically." I was overcome with relief. Jim remained in that hospital for another two weeks before moving to the nearby Brierwood Convalescent Home.

The cheerful manager at Brierwood had instilled a welcoming and compassionate atmosphere, but the reality was grim. It was hard to tell the residents who had only physical infirmities from those with psychiatric illnesses. In truth, all the residents looked to be suffering from a combination of physical pain, psychological depression, and humiliation.

Jim arrived at Brierwood in a wheelchair and with the tube still protruding from his stomach. The tube was eventually removed, but he never gained enough strength to give up the wheelchair. I was able to spend three days visiting with Jim at Brierwood. On the first day, I nervously approached the reception desk and told the attendant that I was there to see Jim. "Oh good," she said, "Just follow me. He's waiting for you in his room." We walked down a narrow corridor, turned a corner, and entered a room. Or, I should say, a tiny alcove containing a bed and little else. This was Jim's so-called room. Beyond the curtain on the far side of the bed were the beds of several other residents. Contrary to our expectations, Jim was obviously not in his room.

As the attendant and I began to search for him, we passed several pajama-clad residents in the corridor, one of whom directed us to an open door. Peering in, I spotted Jim seated in his chair amid shadows and clutter. The room was filled with mattresses, linen shelves, and whirling laundry machines. "Hello, Ron," he said in a low, ironic version of his usual greeting. His embarrassment was a match for my discomfort, as I was shaken by the pathetic circumstances. We had hardly begun to converse, however, when a woman who identified herself as a social worker appeared. Paying no attention whatsoever to Jim, who sat just beside me, and with no preliminary chatter, she asked me directly for my instructions in the event that Jim should die! I could hardly believe my ears. Since I was in no mood to discuss such matters, I angrily dismissed her.

I rolled Jim into the courtyard where the sunlight brightened our spirits and reawakened the brotherly bond. Physically, he looked weak and sickly, but he was surprisingly alert and talkative, especially considering what had just happened. Because we had not had a real conversation since before the episode with NMS, I asked him how he was feeling. He shrugged off the question and showed no inclination to discuss his recent medical experiences. He was coping with the situation on his own terms within his own interior world. He seemed to have friends at

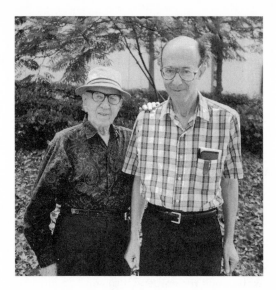

Jim and his father, 1994

Brierwood, or at least acquaintances, because he nodded greetings to several people as we traveled a path around the courtyard. After each acquaintance passed by, he summarized what he knew of them. His clear favorite was a girl in her mid-twenties. She was certainly the prettiest and the most vivacious of all the women we encountered. Jim repeatedly solicited her attention, but she never responded with more than a curt greeting. Something was brewing beneath the surface that I was unable to fathom.

Jim began reminiscing in an uncharacteristic manner. "Yes," he stated, "I enjoyed my life as a graduate student. You may remember, Ron, that my professor asked me to be his teaching assistant. I was honored by his offer because it was well known that only the best students became teaching assistants. I guess the professor liked me. In truth, I knew my stuff, and I think that I could have been a good teacher. Unfortunately, it was precisely at that time that I became ill, so I never got the opportunity to teach. Dad, of course, was a good teacher, and I bet that you are too."

We parked his wheelchair beside by an old orange tree. Dozens of pigeons were fluttering and landing all around us, but Jim paid them little attention as we began discussing authors, covering ground we had covered often before.

"What about Aldous Huxley?" I asked. "You like him don't you?"

"Well, I've read most of his novels, beginning with *Crome Yellow*, his first. And, of course, *Brave New World*. I'm sure you've read that, Ron. You've probably also read his latest, called *Island*, but I have not. From a purely literary standpoint, his finest work is *After a Many Summer Dies the Swan*."

"Oh, really? I'm not familiar with that book."

"I'm surprised that you don't know it, Ron. The main character, a rich guy named Jo Stoyte, is modeled after William Randolph Hearst, the newspaper magnate. You know who Hearst is, don't you? I think you've been up to see his castle near Monterey. Anyway, in the book, the Hearst character combines a life of material decadence with a quest for immortality. It's a superb work, and I recommend it to you."

I pushed Jim's wheelchair through the courtyard at a slow pace as we stopped now and then to chat about literature and other things. Jim tired, though, so I decided it was time for me to leave. He accompanied me to the main entrance of the Brierwood Home where we said our goodbyes. I returned to my motel upset about his physical appearance and perplexed by his unexpected cheerfulness. I avoided thinking about the incident in the laundry room.

Imagine my disappointment when I arrived at the Brierwood Home for my second visit and again Jim could not be found. He was not in his room, and he was not in the laundry room. The attendant asked people if they had seen him, but no one had any suggestions. She then began opening doors at random until we found Jim in a small, totally dark utility room. The situation was pathetic, of course, but also ridiculous, so I chose to make light of it. I guessed right, for his mood quickly brightened, and a few minutes later he offered to show me around the premises. Jim greeted most of the residents we encountered, and introduced me to a few of them.

Full of enthusiasm now, he led me into the kitchen where he introduced me to the chef who was busy preparing lunch. On a patio where tables had been set, Jim and I sat down. An attendant came by serving each of us a plate with potatoes, cooked carrots, and a slice of tough beef. I watched in amazement as Jim picked up the meat in his fingers and began to tear it apart with his teeth. Only then did I notice that while all the other diners had sharp steel knives, we had none. Believing it to be an oversight, I spoke politely to the attendant who left and returned with disposable plastic knives. Later I learned that Jim had been involved in certain "incidents," or fights, one of which was reportedly "over a girl," presumably the young girl I had met. So, the staff had evidently taken the precaution of keeping sharp objects out of Jim's hands. Seeing Jim emaciated and confined to his wheelchair, it was hard to imagine him attacking anyone, but I knew the depths of his depression and anger. As I was also to learn, he did not always take his medications.

Resting in my motel room that evening, I realized that Jim would never return to Castle Hill, so I decided to drive out to Pasadena to pick up his belongings. I arrived at Castle Hill the following morning and asked to see the manager, who quickly retrieved a paper grocery bag which she said contained all his things. Inside, I was dismayed to discover only a dirty pair of pants, a crumpled shirt, a toothbrush, toothpaste, a comb, and a battered copy of a cheap paperback novel. Later, after his death, I experienced a similar surprise when I asked his caretakers at Brierwood for his remaining possessions. They told me that there was nothing of any value: no books, no pictures, no personal papers, and no jewelry; just a few hundred dollars held for him in the office from his accumulated welfare payments. Jim died owning nothing.

I had one more day before flying back to Montreal. I feared that this might be the last time, ever, that I would see my brother and, as things turned out, it was. I suspected that Jim might be thinking similar thoughts, but neither of us even hinted at the possibility when we decided to walk around the block. It may have been the first time that Jim had left the premises since he had arrived at Brierwood some six months earlier, and he clearly enjoyed the change of scenery. We proceeded very slowly through the neighborhood of modest, but well-kept, homes, and we stopped several times to rest and chat. In fact, since I was pushing Jim from behind his wheelchair, we *had* to stop in order to chat, and Jim did want to chat.

Something had made him unusually talkative and animated. It could have been a change in his medication, an awareness of the occasion, or perhaps a combination of the two. Regardless, Jim wanted to reminisce. He spoke about our automobile trip from Chicago to Los Angeles, about the high school we both attended, and once more about his graduate studies at UCLA. He spoke warmly about Mom, and he proudly recalled an incident in which Dad had helped him in a difficult situation. During one of our rest stops, I reported that I had started to read *After a Many Summer Dies the Swan*, the Aldous Huxley novel that he had recommended. He responded with a critique of the book, notwithstanding the fact that at least 35 years had passed since he had last read it. Astonishingly, he recalled not only details of the plot but also the names of all four central characters. He noticed my astonishment at his performance, and he delighted in it.

With sadness in my heart, I returned to Montreal. Although my brother lived another four months, we had only a few telephone conversations after my departure from L.A., and none was reassuring. Several times he even refused to pick up the phone when I called. On other occasions, he would speak to me semi-coherently. The nurses reported that he was not eating and he was refusing to take his medications. Clearly, he was deteriorating both psychologically and physically. When nothing more could be done for him at Brierwood, he was sent to a psychiatric hospital and then transferred to a medical hospital on the following day. It was difficult to get information about his condition. I was told only that Jim was anemic and that there were "complications." Two weeks later, at age 65, he died in Hollywood.

What Happens to People with Schizophrenia through the Years?

As noted earlier, when Emil Kraepelin first described the disease that we now call schizophrenia, he named it dementia praecox. The word *dementia* had been around since ancient Greece. Literally, it means to be out of (*de*) one's mind (*menos*), but its usage in the nineteenth century implied a chronic, incurable deterioration of mental functions. Because *praecox* means premature, Kraepelin was naming a type of premature madness. In addition to the delusions, the hallucinations, and the disorganized thinking that were already considered characteristic of dementia, Kraepelin emphasized the poor prognosis for people with dementia praecox. In his early descriptions, which he later softened, Kraepelin wrote that the disease started early and progressively deteriorated, with no possibility of recovery. Modern critics have noted, however, that his asylum housed only the worst cases, so he probably knew little about individuals who had less severe diseases and who may have fared better. Kraepelin may have been led to an excessively pessimistic conclusion because of the sampling bias in his observations. In any event, schizophrenia, as we know it today, is not really premature and not always deteriorating.

Schizophrenia often begins with an initial psychotic episode, as it did for my brother. Thereafter, the disease follows one of several possible patterns of progression. In developed countries, at least, antipsychotic medications are typically administered soon after the initial episode, and these medications usually cause the positive symptoms to subside. With continuing medication, the symptoms will further stabilize over the following years, but relapses with psychotic manifestations may still occur at irregular intervals. Symptoms, severity of symptoms, and the patient's overall level of functioning all vary considerably from patient to patient.

The idea that a person with schizophrenia can fully recover is controversial. A cure is currently inconceivable, because it would mean eliminating the *causes* of the disease, but treatment strategies that block the underlying causes or that compensate for impairments might restore functions lost to the disease. A report from George W. Bush's New Freedom Commission on Mental Health, in 2002, promoted the concept of recovery in mental health based on the model of Alcoholics Anonymous. The optimistic judgments in the report sparked hope among patients and their families, but overall the approach was viewed as confused and naive by critics. Not everyone believes that recovery is possible, or at least not full recovery, or not in the majority of persons with schizophrenia. Moreover, it is unclear exactly what recovery would look like in schizophrenia.

The widespread use of antipsychotic medications and, to a lesser extent, psychosocial therapies, has undoubtedly improved the lives of people with schizophrenia in the past half century. The drugs have been especially successful in controlling psychotic symptoms and preventing relapses after periods of remission. Yet, on the broader question of whether patients get better or worse over time, and what factors influence the outcome, there is little consensus. What might seem like an easy question turns out to be difficult to answer because there are so many ways to approach it. First, there is the choice of which patients to study: either inpatients or outpatients; either a small number of patients who can be followed from the beginning of their illnesses (prospective studies) or large collections of patients culled from medical records (**retrospective** studies). Next, the choice of a yardstick for measuring improvement: is it an improvement in symptoms, the ability to live independently, physical health, social activity, employment, or a combination of all of these?

To illustrate why it is so difficult to say whether people with schizophrenia can recover, and what exactly that might mean, I will describe two recent studies that reached very different conclusions. In the first study, 1,633 initially psychotic patients were selected for study on the basis of hospital and clinic records; the patients came from 14 culturally diverse, international institutions. Fifteen years after they had first been entered into the records, the patients were assessed on a variety of criteria including symptoms, functional abilities, social interactions, and residential status. The data reveal that about 50 percent of the patients had "recovered" and about 40 percent had not had any psychotic episodes in the most recent two years. Forty-six percent had worked for pay for most of the previous two years, and an additional 28 percent had done unpaid housework. The authors conclude, "The overarching message of [this study] is that schizophrenia and related psychoses are best seen developmentally as episodic disorders with a rather favorable outcome for a significant proportion of patients."[1]

Quite a different picture emerges from a second study. Here, 6,642 outpatients in 10 European countries were assessed during three years of antipsychotic drug treatment. The investigators used three criteria for improvement: reduced symptoms; good "quality of life"; and functional competence, meaning ability to engage in work activities, social interactions, and everyday chores such as shopping, housekeeping, and paying bills. A patient was scored as being in remission if he or she met one or more of the criteria for a minimum of two years, including the final year of the study (year 3). Thirty-three percent of the patients experienced a remission as measured by a reduction of symptoms; 13 percent had remissions according to the functional criterion; and 27 percent had remissions as judged by the quality of life. However, when recovery was defined as having achieved all three criteria (symptoms, functions, and quality of life), only 4 percent were found to be recovered. In contrast to the conclusion drawn in the study described above, the authors of this study wrote, "When using a stringent definition of recovery based on objective outcomes, a very low proportion of patients with schizophrenia who start antipsychotic treatment achieve recovery."[2]

Faced with such seemingly contradictory conclusions, two investigators reviewed the literature on outcomes in schizophrenia to see if the data show any overall consensus. Rather than focusing on rates of "recovery," the researchers boiled down all the results into two basic categories of outcomes: good and bad. They examined data from 18 independent studies, all of which were of the prospective type, that is, the

patients were selected for the studies as soon as they had been diagnosed with schizophrenia. For their review, the investigators computed
the percentages of good and bad outcomes in each study, while ignoring
differences in how good outcomes and poor outcomes had been defined.
They found that good outcomes varied between approximately 20 and
55 percent and poor outcomes varied between approximately 7 and 60
percent. Thus, not only did the results vary greatly from one study to
the next, but *neither* good outcomes *nor* poor outcomes predominated.
In all but 1 of the 18 studies, a large proportion of the patients were not
placed in either category, presumably because their diseases progressed
as a mix of the good and the bad. The authors of the review conclude
that it is impossible to generalize because "the course and outcome of
schizophrenia is characterised by mainly unexplained heterogeneity
rather than uniform poor outcome."[3]

The studies summarized in the preceding paragraphs highlight the
highly diverse nature of outcomes for people who have schizophrenia.
While understandably troubling for patients and for the families of
patients, this heterogeneity of symptoms over time can be taken as
further evidence for the heterogeneity of the disease itself. It would be
reasonable to infer that the different outcomes are associated with different subtypes of schizophrenia. If the subtypes can be defined by
genetic or other biological criteria, and matched with various courses of
the disease, it should be possible to predict outcomes. Meanwhile, researchers have identified a few factors, unrelated to diagnosis, that associate with good outcomes. It is clear that favorable outcomes are most
likely when the initial psychotic episode is short in duration and comes
relatively late in life. Also, not surprisingly, patients who avoid substance abuse and regularly take their medications do better than those
who abuse drugs or neglect their medications. And, again as one would
expect, the long-range outlook is best for patients who have the least
amount of psychosis during the first two years of their illnesses or who
have generally mild symptoms. For the most part, these findings suggest that those patients with the milder forms of the disease have the
best chance of a favorable long-term course.

One further point about the course of schizophrenia is worth noting.
Because there are virtually no untreated patients with schizophrenia to

be found in modern psychiatric investigations, the data on outcomes pertain only to patients taking antipsychotic drugs and receiving supportive care. The natural course of the untreated disease is unknown, or at least is not described in the professional literature.

The prospect of increasing the chances of a good outcome through active intervention has generated great interest. Can professional caretakers adopt practical measures that will make remission or recovery more likely? One promising idea focuses on providing intensive psychological and social support as early as possible after the patient's initial psychotic episode, in addition to administering antipsychotic medication. In projects of this type, each patient is typically coupled with a professional caregiver who is responsible for the patient's mental health and general welfare. The caregiver maintains contact with the patient, provides psychological support, and coordinates all services appropriate for the patient. The patients are offered training in social skills and problem solving, and are advised on strategies to cope with symptoms. Family members are asked to participate in the treatment program. Lastly, the programs emphasize the importance of taking medications as prescribed.

Some researchers have reported good results with early intervention programs of this type. That is, symptoms apparently lessen, social and vocational activities increase, and remissions last longer. However, at least one study raises doubts about the effectiveness of early interventions.[4] The study followed a rigorous research design, as required in any examination of a new treatment option. First, two groups of patients were randomly assigned to either the experimental group, which received early interventions, or the comparison group, which received standard treatments at a community mental health center. Second, the assessments of the patients' mental health status were done by professionals who did not know which group the patients had been assigned to (so-called blind assessments). Third, and importantly, the long-term effects of the treatment were investigated. Patients were assessed two years after the treatments (experimental and standard) and then again after five years.

When the effects of intensive early intervention were assessed two years after they started, the investigators found statistically significant benefits on measures of negative symptoms, psychotic symptoms, and "global functioning." However, these same benefits were not evident after five years, implying that they had worn off. For other measures of early intervention, covering substance abuse, depression, and suicidal behavior, there was no effect even at two years. Although these findings are disappointing, it is possible that longer lasting benefits of early intervention might be achieved by either extending the length of the intensive treatment period or adjusting other aspects of the program. Helping patients to keep up with their medications—called *compliance*— is one important means by which early interventions might promote good outcomes.

Compliance is the elephant in the schizophrenia recovery room. Numerous studies have shown that noncompliance is strongly associated with relapses, hospitalizations, attempted suicides, and generally poor outcomes. Researchers find that the rates of noncompliance range from 20 to 56 percent, depending on the clinical setting, the patient population, and the duration of observation. In a recent study of 6,731 patients undergoing outpatient treatment, 29 percent were noncompliant.[5] These high rates of noncompliance represent a serious problem for which there is no easy solution. While all psychiatric professionals recognize the risks associated with noncompliance, the patients themselves may have less understanding of the risks or be less concerned about them. And yet it is the patients themselves who decide whether or not to take the drugs.[6] The main factors associated with noncompliance are alcohol and substance abuse, independent living, and severe symptoms. It has been suggested that strategies to encourage compliance should be targeted to patients in these high-risk groups, but given the nature of the risk factors, that will not be easy.

Death marks the final insult for people who have schizophrenia, and for the majority it comes far too early. It seems not to matter whether an individual has severe symptoms or mild symptoms, many remissions or few remissions: most die early. A team of epidemiologists examined the results from 37 previous studies, each of which had calculated a mortality rate for people with schizophrenia and compared it with the rate for people in the general population who were matched with the patients for age and sex. The authors concluded that people with schizophrenia, of whatever age or sex, have two or three times the risk of dying as people in the general population.[7] On average, people with schizophrenia live approximately 15 to 20 fewer years than people in the general population. Furthermore, and disturbingly, the gap between mortality rates in the schizophrenia population and in the general population increased during the final three decades of the twentieth century. The reasons for the gap and its apparent widening are not well understood, but many factors are likely involved.

Suicide is a major cause of early death for people with schizophrenia. In the epidemiological study mentioned above, people with schizophrenia were nearly 13 times more likely to die of suicide than were people of equivalent age and sex in the general population. Overall, about 5 percent of people with schizophrenia die of suicide, usually near the onset of their disease; the comparable figure for the general population is about 0.012 percent. By contrast, more than 50 percent of people with schizophrenia die of cardiovascular disease. Digestive diseases, infectious diseases, and respiratory diseases are also more common among people with schizophrenia than in the general population. There are many explanations for the high rates of disease among people with schizophrenia. The lifestyles of people who have schizophrenia—typically involving heavy smoking, little exercise, poor diet, and limited access to health care services—are a contributing factor. In addition, the very medications that improve the patients' behavioral symptoms may damage their physical health.

Controversy surrounds the role of antipsychotic medications in the premature deaths of people who have schizophrenia. Different studies have given different results, in large part owing to the problem of finding enough patients for the control group, that is, finding patients who have not taken antipsychotic medications. In my brother's case, I have little doubt that the drugs contributed to his death at the relatively young age of 65. The neuroleptic malignant syndrome, which he probably had, disrupts several major body systems, and it can be fatal if not treated quickly and appropriately. Fortunately, in the years since Jim succumbed to the consequences of NMS, a better awareness of the danger has reduced both the incidence of NMS and the number of deaths resulting from it. Also, the second-generation antipsychotics are less likely to produce NMS, and the preferential use of these newer drugs has reduced the risk. Although the second-generation antipsychotics are relatively safe with respect to NMS, they may nonetheless contribute to premature deaths through other adverse effects, among which are the increased risk of seizures, the reduction of white blood cell numbers, and a complex condition known as metabolic syndrome, which involves weight gain, diabetes, and cardiovascular disease.

SUMMARY

- Contrary to what people previously believed, schizophrenia is not a disease that inevitably leads to progressive deterioration. The lifetime course is highly variable, and most patients have periods of remission in which symptoms decline in severity or completely disappear. However, psychotic relapses are common, and true recovery is rare.
- If the first psychotic episode comes at a relatively young age and is brief, then the outcome is more likely to be good. Also, patients tend to have longer periods of remission if their symptoms are relatively mild, if they avoid substance abuse, and if they take their medications as prescribed.
- Some research suggests that programs of intensive treatment implemented shortly after the first psychotic episode lead to better outcomes. However, the effect may be short-lived. In one study, a benefit of early interventions was found when tests of symptoms and everyday functioning were conducted two years after the onset of treatment, but after five years the beneficial effects had disappeared.
- People with schizophrenia commonly suffer from poor physical health, and the average life of a schizophrenia patient is 15 to 20 years shorter than for someone in the general population. People with schizophrenia are 13 times more likely to commit suicide than are people in the general population.

21

Reflections

Strangely, my parents never spoke the s-word, never said that my brother had schizophrenia. Despite their reticence, schizophrenia was the disease that defined his life, if not his person. If it had not been for schizophrenia, he probably would have been a teacher and a scholar, but with the disease, he struggled just to stay out of hospitals. Instead of enjoying the rewards of a productive career and the love of his children, he suffered frustration, anger, and psychological turmoil. In the midst of all of that, I am proud to say, he was comforted by the love of his brother and parents. Even in the worst of times and even when he shunned us, I know that he drew strength from us.

I could not have written this book—nor would I have written it—if I did not have fond memories of the times we spent together. Unfortunately, there was a lot of sadness too, especially in the final year of Jim's life. Beginning with the neuroleptic malignant syndrome, he suffered a downward spiral from which he was unable to escape. In telling Jim's story here, I have had to keep an emotional distance from the facts. The reader will know, however, that reliving some of the events has been painful, none more so than those of Jim's final days.

Inevitably, a disease like schizophrenia affects not only the victim but also the lives of those close to the victim. My mother died 18 years ahead of Jim, so at least she was spared his awful death. However, she suffered dearly from disappointment and sadness. Despite my own enthusiasm for neuroscience, which I conveyed to her, she never deviated from her psychological interpretation of schizophrenia, and I think it was for this reason that she could not completely shed the burden of guilt. Dad, too, died before Jim did, although just one year earlier. He had continued to hope for so long that when he was finally forced to accept the permanence of Jim's handicap, his sadness was profound. But Dad was stoic by nature and by resolve, so he did his best to hide his feelings. So far as I could tell, he viewed Jim's illness neither from a strictly psychological perspective nor from a neuroscientific perspective. I think it was all a muddle for him, and I think he preferred it that way. No theory could restore to Jim the fullness of life that my father had wanted for him.

As for myself, I grieve for Jim and I miss him. In the early days, before his illness, we had fun together, and I learned much from him. Later, even though we lived far apart, we stayed connected in a special, brotherly way. When I visited him and he was feeling well, we could still enjoy each other's company; and on the other occasions, at least I was there for him. All along, I searched for answers, and I gradually found them in science.

I sometimes reflect on whether Jim's life would have turned out differently had he been 24 years old today and just now experiencing his first psychotic episode. In most respects, I think not, because little has changed in the treatment and management of schizophrenia during the past 50-plus years. If he became ill today, he would probably not be given the shock treatments he got then, but the drugs would be similar to, and about as effective as, the chlorpromazine that he began taking in 1960. Which is to say that his positive symptoms (paranoia, confusion) would be suppressed to about the same extent, and his negative symptoms (social withdrawal, low motivation) would be persistent. He would probably still live in some type of board-and-care residence and still require hospitalization during relapses. However, because the state of California has ended its program of generous financial support, I would be paying his rent and living expenses. Some of his former co-residents would now be homeless and quite likely would not be taking prescribed medications. As a consequence, these unfortunate people would be susceptible to drug abuse, ongoing psychosis, and violence. Only the end of Jim's life would be significantly different, I believe, and that is because precautions would be taken to prevent neuroleptic malignant syndrome. I cannot say how, exactly, he would live out his final years if they were to occur in the twenty-first century, but I am fairly certain that he would suffer less than he did.

Whereas the reality of life with schizophrenia has not changed much since Jim became ill, the way in which people perceive the disease has changed considerably. When Jim's symptoms first appeared, the fundamental nature of schizophrenia, and indeed of all the major mental illnesses, was poorly understood and widely debated. Some people opted for a psychological interpretation, and others suspected a neurobiological basis. Opinions shifted toward a neuroscientific interpretation after the development of antipsychotic medications and the popularization of mood-altering and other psychoactive drugs, because these products provided dramatic evidence of mind control by physical means. If a pill could calm a psychotic rage or lift a dark depression, then surely these so-called mental disorders must actually be disorders of the brain. And so the physical approach to mental illness began to replace the fantasies of psychoanalysis and the half-baked ideas of certain social commentators.[1] As a result, I presume, families today face less guilt, fear, and confusion than our family experienced.

Epilogue

The rapid collapse of psychoanalysis in the latter half of the twentieth century found its counterpart in the spectacular rise of scientific knowledge about the human brain.[1] Research into the structure and function of the brain is driven not only by medical interests, including the concerns of psychiatry, but also by basic curiosity. Now, the winds of hope are driving an ever quickening pace of research into schizophrenia. As we wait for this research to bear fruit, we should not lose sight of the needs of current patients. We must ensure that they get the compassionate support that they deserve, which means, of course, finding the money to pay for the services. So, how can we best allocate public resources between programs for the maintenance and treatment of patients and programs in support of the thriving research effort? It is a problem faced by both policy makers and charitable donors, and I have no absolute solution. However, I believe that the following assessment by a group of psychiatric scholars accurately sums up the situation:

> Many people with schizophrenia have persisting symptoms, despite the best mix of interventions we can offer. . . . For schizophrenia, with the current mix of interventions we can only reduce 13 percent of the burden. If we improve efficiencies within the current services, we can do somewhat better (22 percent). In a utopian world, even if unlimited funding were available [for services], three-quarters of the burden of schizophrenia would remain unavoidable. This is a powerful argument for investing in applied and basic research.[2]

The reputation of science is built on its record of success in finding answers to problems in the physical world. Because schizophrenia essentially involves a problem with a physical thing, the brain, it is subject to all the power and precision of science. Knowing this, we can take heart in a pronouncement from the editors of *Nature* magazine: "There are many ways in which the understanding and treatment of conditions such as schizophrenia are ripe for a revolution."[3]

While I agree that our *understanding* of schizophrenia is "ripe for a revolution," I do not expect that the *treatment* of schizophrenia will ripen in revolutionary ways any time soon. Earlier in this book, I wrote that no new physical therapy or any new method of social therapy is likely to significantly enhance current treatment options. Moreover, the development of new, more effective drugs is challenged by the complexity of neurobiological defects in schizophrenia. The director of the U.S. National Institute of Mental Health, Dr. Thomas Insel, noted in October 2012 that "the private sector seems infected with a misguided sense of doom and gloom for research and development."[4] Eventually, though, the science of molecular genetics, meaning the study of DNA, will produce results. Looking far into the future, it is conceivable that genetic manipulations could provide total protection against the risk of schizophrenia and a complete cure if prevention fails. In the shorter term, and more likely, genetics can become a useful tool in the service of existing treatment programs.

A perfect solution would be to correct, at an early age or even before birth, the gene mutations that create the risk of schizophrenia. Gene therapies have been successfully tested in animal models, and human trials have begun. Several techniques are used. Most commonly, a normal gene is inserted into the genome to replace the mutated gene. It is also possible, in some cases, to undo or reverse the mutation by attacking it with special chemicals. Other options include activating alternative copies of the mutated gene and activating a healthy gene that functions in a manner similar to the mutated gene. Unfortunately, despite the appeal of these molecular tools, their application to complex diseases like schizophrenia is not straightforward. Recall that a patient with schizophrenia may have a very large number of mutant genes. Scientists are currently challenged to replace or correct just *one* mutant gene. If it were actually necessary to correct hundreds or thousands of mutations, the task would be so formidable that gene therapy for schizophrenia would have to be ruled out. On the other hand, it might turn out that correcting just one or two key genes would be sufficient.

An effective treatment might also be implemented not by correcting any mutant genes but instead by targeting the functional defects created by the mutant genes. Even if many genes are involved in creating the risk for schizophrenia, they may all contribute to a single defect in the brain. Discovering the functions of the proteins that genes make can be as difficult as discovering the risk genes themselves—or more so. Nevertheless, imagine a scenario in which all the risk genes for schizophrenia make proteins required for synaptic communication.

Effective communication between pairs of synapsing neurons requires a complex machinery, which, in turn, requires a variety of proteins. Tiny extensions of the two participating neurons must be built in such a manner that each extension lies precisely parallel to the other across a gap of less than one-thousandth of a human hair. The sending neuron must have membrane channels that can generate rapid voltage changes (action potentials); it must make the neurotransmitter substance; and it must be able to recruit and release sufficient amounts of the neurotransmitter in conjunction with its action potentials. The receiving neuron has its own set of specializations centered on detecting and responding to the neurotransmitter.

My description of synapses is simplified, and my suggestion that all the risk genes make proteins that are necessary for normal synaptic communication is probably not correct, but consider the implications if it were true: a single drug might be able to compensate for all the genetic errors simply by boosting the efficiency of synapses. For example, an effective drug might increase the ability of the receiving neurons to detect the transmitter substance.

Genetic screening to identify people at risk for schizophrenia is another likely application of current research. Screening for genes that confer the risk of disease is becoming increasingly common for a variety of disorders, including Tay Sachs disease, Huntington's disease, and cystic fibrosis. However, all the foregoing disorders are relatively easy to screen for because they involve single gene mutations. A geneticist needs only to examine that one gene to determine whether the person will get the disease. By contrast, numerous genes are associated with schizophrenia, and the list is not yet complete, so no single gene and no group of specified genes is predictive of schizophrenia. (The low predictive value of known risk genes is discussed in chapter 4.) Nevertheless, our ability to identify people at risk will grow as our knowledge of genetics increases, and eventually genetic screens will provide an acceptable degree of reliability.

Once appropriate screens become available, people at risk can be monitored to detect abnormalities in brain development (using imaging technologies) and cognitive function (using psychological tests). If problems are detected early enough, therapeutic interventions can be started before overt symptoms appear, and further development of the disease could be blocked. A potential drawback to genetic screening is the anxiety of family members after positive findings. Therefore, the efficacy of treatments must keep pace with the accuracy of genetic screening. One way this could happen is by using our knowledge of genetics to personalize medications.

Dozens of drugs are currently licensed for use with schizophrenia, but psychiatrists are given little guidance as to which drug or which combination of drugs will work best for individual patients. The same drug can produce different effects in different patients. For example, a drug may relieve symptoms and cause few side effects in one patient, but in another patient the same drug may have little beneficial effect and produce significant adverse effects. A second drug might have completely different effects in the same two patients, and so on. Findings such as these have prompted the suggestion that the varied responses to antipsychotic drugs might reflect different schizophrenia subtypes.[5]

Earlier, I mentioned other evidence for schizophrenia subtypes, including differences in symptoms. Many, if not all, of these observable distinctions probably result from differences in DNA. It would not be surprising to learn that there is a molecular signature for each subtype. One constellation of gene variants will produce one subtype of schizophrenia, and another constellation of genes will produce a different subtype. If this turns out to be true, we would have a sound scientific basis for personalizing medications. Once the gene profile for a particular subtype has been determined, and the protein products of these genes identified, it becomes possible to select drugs with relevant actions, or even to design new drugs with the desired specificity. The appropriate drug might be selected to block a specific protein in some cases and substitute for it in other cases.

This strategy is already beginning to pay off in the treatment of cancers. The gastrointestinal stromal tumors, for example, are highly resistant to chemotherapy and therefore very dangerous. However, a subset of patients can be effectively treated with a drug that inhibits a particular enzyme; these patients, and only these patients, have a mutation in a gene that makes a protein that is targeted by the enzyme. The same mutation is found in a subset of patients with lung cancers; again, patients with the mutation respond well to the enzyme-inhibiting drug, while other patients who have no mutation in this specific gene do not respond. Another example relates to a gene called *ERBB2*, which is abnormally represented by extra copies in about 30 percent of people with breast cancer. Once these people are identified, they are given a drug, trastuzumab (marketed as Herceptin), that interferes with the protein product of *ERBB2*. Herceptin is highly effective in people with the amplified *ERBB2* gene, but it is useless in people with breast cancer who have the normal two copies of the gene.

Two thousand years ago, people believed the world to be flat, they knew nothing of electricity, and they thought that mental illness was due to bad body fluids. Later, people found that they could navigate around the earth, they invented computers, and they began to investigate the brain. In the mid-twentieth century, a drug was discovered that could suppress the worst symptoms of schizophrenia. Slowly, but progressively, we gather knowledge about all things relevant to schizophrenia: the genes that cause it, the environments that influence it, its neurodevelopmental defects, and its underlying brain mechanisms. As we look to the future, we must be patient. New discoveries will answer more of our questions. Although some advances will not come quickly enough to improve the lives of people who now have the disease, in the long run science will defeat schizophrenia.

Notes

Prologue

1. All data are from PubMed, the online database maintained by the United States National Library of Science.

Chapter 2. Who Gets Schizophrenia and Why?

1. J. McGrath et al. (2008). Schizophrenia: A concise overview of incidence, prevalence, and mortality. *Epidemiologic Reviews* 30:67–76.

2. The estimate given here is called the *lifetime morbid risk*. For definitions of other types of prevalence measures, see the glossary.

3. The geneticist Irving Gottesman provides a full account of family, adoption, and twin studies in his book *Schizophrenia Genesis: The Origins of Madness* (1991). New York: W. H. Freeman.

4. P. Tienari et al. (2004). Genotype-environment interaction in schizophrenia-spectrum disorder: Long-term follow-up study of Finnish adoptees. *British Journal of Psychiatry* 184:216–222.

5. On average, 50 percent of the genes are shared between pairs of dizygotic twins; individual pairs may share more than half or fewer than half of their genes. Also, strictly speaking, it is not the genes that are identical but the alleles.

6. A full description of these early twin studies is found in Gottesman 1991.

7. A. G. Cardno and I. I. Gottesman (2000). Twin studies of schizophrenia: From bow-and-arrow concordances to star wars and Mx functional genomics. *American Journal of Medical Genetics* 97:12–17.

8. I use the 50 percent concordance rate for identical twins as the realistic approximation of a rate for which there is a range of estimates. My interpretations of the twin studies would be no different if the concordance were 46 percent or 61 percent or some other number near 50 percent.

9. For a scientific discussion, see P. M. Visscher, W. G. Hill, and N. R. Wray (2008). Heritability in the genomics era—concepts and misconceptions. *Nature Reviews, Genetics* 9:255–266.

Chapter 4. Which Genes Cause Schizophrenia?

1. The definition of a gene has changed as its properties have become known in greater detail. For a current, molecular, definition see the glossary.

2. The prediction depends on whether the healthy parent possesses ("carries") one or no mutated copies of the recessive gene; the diseased parent always possesses two mutated copies.

3. All percentage values are taken from I. I. Gottesman (1991). *Schizophrenia Genesis: The Origins of Madness*. New York: W. H. Freeman.

4. The International Schizophrenia Consortium (2009). Common polygenic variation contributes to risk of schizophrenia and bipolar disease. *Nature* 460: 748–752.

5. P. F. Sullivan, M. J. Daly, and M. O'Donovan (2012). Genetic architectures of psychiatric disorders: The emerging picture and its implications. *Nature Reviews Genetics* 13:537–551.

6. Strictly speaking, it is incorrect to say that a certain *gene* creates a risk for schizophrenia (or any other disease). Rather, it is a *variant* of the gene that confers the risk.

7. Here and elsewhere, when I refer to gene "activity," I mean the process whereby genes (DNA) make ribonucleic acid (**RNA**), which later makes protein. The technical term for the production of RNA from DNA is *gene expression*.

8. For discussion on whether schizophrenia is a single disease, see chapter 16.

9. H. L. Allen et al. (2010). Hundreds of variants clustered in genomic loci and biological pathways affect human height. *Nature* 467:832–838.

10. Although I say that 180 "genes" were identified, it is actually the case that 180 "single nucleotide polymorphisms" (also known as SNPs, "snips," or "loci") were identified. SNPs are variants of the single DNA "letters" that make up the genetic code. Some of the SNPs are in the protein-coding regions of the DNA (exons), while others are in the regulatory regions (introns).

11. B. Maher (2008). The case of the missing heritability. *Nature* 456:18–21.

12. J. A. Tennessen et al. (2012). Evolution and functional impact of rare coding variation from deep sequencing of human exomes. *Science* 337:64–69.

13. M. Lynch (2010). Rate, molecular spectrum, and consequences of human mutation. *Proceedings of the National Academy of Sciences USA* 107:961–968. Quote on p. 966.

14. B. E. Bernstein et al. (2012). An integrated encyclopedia of DNA elements in the human genome. *Nature* 489:57–74; M. T. Maurano et al. (2012). Systematic localization of common disease-associated variation in regulatory DNA. *Science* 337:1190–1195.

15. J. T. Glessner et al. (2010). Strong synaptic transmission impact by copy number variations in schizophrenia. *Proceedings of the National Academy of Sciences USA* 107:10584–10589.

16. A. Petronis (2010). Epigenetics as a unifying principle in the aetiology of complex traits and diseases. *Nature* 465:721–727.

17. For more discussion of results and strategies in current genetic research, see E. S. Gershon, N. Alliey-Rodriguez, and C. Liu (2011). After GWAS: Searching for genetic risk for schizophrenia and bipolar disorder. *American Journal of Psychiatry* 168:256–256. (The abbreviation GWAS stands for genome-wide association study.)

Chapter 5. A Consultation with Dr. Held (1957)

1. E. Shorter (1997). *A History of Psychiatry: From the Era of the Asylum to the Age of Prozac.* New York: John Wiley & Sons.

2. Both quotations from Shorter 1997, pp. 174–175.

3. F. Fromm-Reichman (1952). Some aspects of psychoanalytic psychotherapy with schizophrenics. In E. B. Brody and F. C. Redlich, eds., *Psychotherapy with Schizophrenics.* New York: International Universities Press, pp. 89–111. Quote on p. 90.

4. F. Fromm-Reichman (1948). Notes on the development of treatment of schizophrenics by psychoanalytic psychotherapy. *Psychiatry* 11:263–273. Quote on p. 265.

5. The comment of John Neill is quoted by Shorter 1997, p. 177.

Chapter 6. Which Aspects of the Environment Cause Schizophrenia?

1. The involvement of both genetic and environmental causes is highlighted in Tanya Marie Luhrmann's essay, Beyond the brain, *Wilson Quarterly,* summer 2012:28–34.

2. S. L. Matheson et al. (2011). A systematic meta-review grading the evidence for non-genetic risk factors and putative antecedents of schizophrenia. *Schizophrenia Research* 133:133–142.

3. A. Kong et al. (2012). Rate of *de novo* mutations and the importance of father's age to disease risk. *Nature* 488:471–475.

4. P. Casadio et al. (2011). Cannabis use in young people: The risk for schizophrenia. *Neuroscience and Biobehavioral Reviews* 35:1779–1787.

5. A. S. Brown and D. J. Derkits (2010). Prenatal infection and schizophrenia: A review of epidemiologic and translational studies. *American Journal of Psychiatry* 167:261–280.

6. S. Arieti (1974). An overview of schizophrenia from a predominately psychological approach. *American Journal of Psychiatry* 131:241–249. Quote on p. 342.

7. M. J. Goldstein (1987). The UCLA high-risk project. *Schizophrenia Bulletin* 13:505–514.

8. J. F. Dunn and R. Plomin (1990). *Separate Lives: Why Siblings Are So Different*. New York: Basic Books.

9. E. Turkheimer and M. Waldron (2000). Nonshared environment: A theoretical, methodological, and quantitative review. *Psychological Bulletin* 126:78–108.

10. Matheson et al. 2011.

11. T. D. Cannon et al. (2008). Prediction of psychosis in youth at high clinical risk. *Archives of General Psychiatry* 65:28–37. Individuals who had sought treatment were interviewed, evaluated, and then followed for another 2.5 years. Overall, the predictions of psychosis were 79 percent accurate.

Chapter 8. Why Does Schizophrenia Begin in Late Adolescence?

1. D. R. Weinberger (1987). Implications of normal brain development for the pathogenesis of schizophrenia. *Archives of General Psychiatry* 44:680–669.

2. As noted earlier, some reports observe subtle signs of abnormality (low intelligence and retarded or incomplete motor skills) in some individuals many years before they become schizophrenic.

3. T. Paus, M. Keshavan, and J. N. Giedd (2008). Why do many psychiatric disorders emerge during adolescence? *Nature Reviews Neuroscience* 9:947–957.

4. M. R. Asato et al. (2010). White matter development in adolescence: A DTI study. *Cerebral Cortex* 20:2122–2131.

5. The hypothesis is updated in D. A. Lewis and P. Levitt (2005). Schizophrenia as a disorder of neurodevelopment. *Annual Review of Neuroscience* 25:409–432. See also, J. L. Rapoport, J. N. Giedd, and N. Gogtay (2012). Neurodevelopmental model of schizophrenia: Update 2012. *Molecular Psychiatry* 17:1228–1238.

6. A. M. McIntosh et al. (2011). Longitudinal volume reductions in people at high genetic risk of schizophrenia as they develop psychosis. *Biological Psychiatry* 69:953–958.

7. A. Hodges et al. (1999). People at risk of schizophrenia: Sample characteristics of the first 100 cases in the Edinburgh High-Risk Study. *British Journal of Psychiatry* 174:547–553. The quote is on p. 548.

8. K. J. Brennand et al. (2011). Modelling schizophrenia using human induced pluripotent stem cells. *Nature* 473:221–225.

9. H. Häfner et al. (1998). Causes and consequences of the gender difference in age at onset of schizophrenia. *Schizophrenia Bulletin* 24:99–113.

Chapter 9. Two State Hospitals (1959–1960)

1. The statement is attributed to Harold Palmer and quoted in P. R. A. May (1968). *Treatment of Schizophrenia: A Comparative Study of Five Treatment Methods*. New York: Science House, p. 51.

2. A full description of the project will be found in May 1968.

3. Quotes from May 1968, pp. 258, 262, and 267.

Chapter 10. What Are the Treatment Options?

1. Although it is generally believed that schizophrenia is a *complex disease* with no single cause, some researchers have proposed that a bacterium, a virus, or another kind of microorganism could play a pivotal role. If true, it is conceivable that a magic bullet could target and nullify the harmful agent. Some researchers claim that the parasite *Toxoplasma gondii* is one such microorganism. At present, however, the evidence for any biological agent acting in this manner is weak.

2. E. Shorter and D. Healy (2007). *Shock Therapy: A History of Electroconvulsive Treatment in Mental Illness*. New Brunswick, NJ: Rutgers Univ. Press. Quote on p. 4.

3. This turned out to be untrue.

4. The account, from Meduna's autobiography, is quoted in E. Shorter (1997). *A History of Psychiatry: From the Era of the Asylum to the Age of Prozac*. New York: John Wiley & Sons, p. 216.

5. Shorter and Healy 2007, p. 298.

6. The story of chlorpromazine's discovery is told in D. Healy (2002). *The Creation of Psychopharmacology*. Cambridge, MA: Harvard Univ. Press.

7. Healy 2002. Quote on p. 89.

8. For a complete list, see table 2 in R. Tandon, H. A. Nasrallah, and M. S. Keshavan (2010). Schizophrenia, "Just the facts" 5. Treatment and prevention past, present and future. *Schizophrenia Research* 122:1–23.

9. Tandon, Nasrallah, and Keshavan 2010, table 5.

10. Tanya Marie Luhrmann (2012). Beyond the brain. *Wilson Quarterly*, summer: 28–34. Quote on p. 33.

11. The quoted evaluation is from Tandon, Nasrallah, and Keshavan 2010, p. 8.

12. The company, Posit Science, was founded by Dr. Michael Merzenich, professor at the University of California, San Francisco. See E. C. Hayden (2012). Game on. *Nature* 483:24–26.

13. M. Girón et al. (2010). Efficacy and effectiveness of individual family intervention on social and clinical functioning and family burden in severe schizophrenia: A 2-year randomized controlled study. *Psychological Medicine* 40:73–84. Quote on p. 81.

Chapter 12. Is Mental Illness in the Mind or in the Brain?

1. R. Descartes (1637, 1965). *Discourse on the Method*, part IV. *A Discourse on Method and Other Works*. J. Epstein, ed. New York: Washington Square Press. Writing in French, Descartes used the word, *l'âme*, which ordinarily translates as

the soul, but his concept of the soul closely resembles our contemporary concept of the mind, so one can legitimately read Descartes as though he were writing about the mind. Also, in these passages Descartes uses forms of the verb *penser* (to think), but it is clear from the entirety of his writings that he is referring to all conscious content.

2. For more on Descartes's ideas and their refutation, see R. Chase (2012). *The Physical Basis of Mental Illness*. Piscataway, NJ: Transaction.

3. Hippocrates, *On the Sacred Disease*, http://classics.mit.edu/Hippocrates /sacred.html. Although attributed to Hippocrates, the text may have been written by one of his students.

4. T. S. Szasz (1961). *The Myth of Mental Illness: Foundations of a Theory of Personal Conduct*. New York: Hoeber-Harper.

5. T. S. Szasz (1976). *Schizophrenia: The Sacred Symbol of Psychiatry*. New York: Basic Books. Quote on p. 105.

6. Ventricular volume and gray matter thickness are examples of *endophenotypes*, biomarkers that lie along the causative pathway between genes and an observable trait or illness. See I. I. Gottesman and T. D. Gould (2003). The endophenotype concept in psychiatry: Etymology and strategic intentions. *American Journal of Psychiatry* 160:636–645.

7. T. Sigurdsson et al. (2010). Impaired hippocampal-prefrontal synchrony in a genetic mouse model of schizophrenia. *Nature* 464:763–767.

8. D. D. Dickerson, A. R. Wolff, and D. K. Bilkey (2010). Abnormal long-range synchrony in a maternal immune activation animal model of schizophrenia. *Journal of Neuroscience* 30:12424–12431.

9. In some studies, the proteins themselves are measured, whereas in other studies the RNAs that make the proteins are measured.

10. D. Arion et al. (2007). Molecular evidence for increased expression of genes related to immune and chaperone function in the prefrontal cortex in schizophrenia. *Biological Psychiatry* 62:711–721.

11. J. E. Lisman et al. (2008). Circuit-based framework for understanding neurotransmitter and risk gene interactions in schizophrenia. *Trends in Neuroscience* 31:234–242.

12. There are four types of glutamate receptors. The alterations of glutamate neurotransmission that are cited in this paragraph all involve the N-methyl-D-aspartate (NMDA) type. For details of pertinent studies, see Lisman et al. 2008.

13. Also, some research suggests that GABA deficits are present only in a subset of schizophrenia patients. See D. W. Volk et al. (2012). Deficits in transcriptional regulators of cortical parvalbumin neurons in schizophrenia. *American Journal of Psychiatry* 169:1082–1091.

14. O. Yizhar et al. (2011). Neocortical excitation/inhibition balance in information processing and social dysfunction. *Nature* 477:171–178.

15. J. E. Belforte et al. (2010). Postnatal NMDA receptor ablation in cortico-limbic interneurons confers schizophrenia-like phenotypes. *Nature Neuroscience* 13:76–83. Note that my summary of this article is simplified. In particular, I refer to a partial elimination of glutamate receptors, whereas actually just one specific type of glutamate receptor, the NMDA receptor, was partially eliminated. Also, I do not mention any effect of the manipulation on the pyramidal cells' responses to glutamate; evidently, the pyramidal cells are much less sensitive to the partial loss of NMDA receptors than are the interneurons, for unknown reasons. The general conclusions are unaffected by my simplifications.

16. The prefrontal cortex is closely tied to *working memory*, which holds thoughts and perceptions just long enough to enable decisions and judgments.

17. Lisman et al. 2008, quote on p. 238.

Chapter 13. The Villa and the Ambassador (1982)

1. The figures are from E. F. Torrey (1997). *Out of the Shadows: Confronting America's Mental Illness Crisis*. New York: John Wiley & Sons. In this book, the author argues forcibly against the policy of deinstitutionalization. Citing, among other factors, the rise in homelessness and the obstacles to obtaining effective treatment in the community, he advocates involuntary hospitalizations as the humane alternative in severe cases.

2. Shirley Star, quoted in B. G. Link et al. (1999). Public conceptions of mental illness: Labels, causes, dangerousness, and social distance. *American Journal of Public Health* 89:1328–1333. Quote on p. 1331.

Chapter 14. Why Is Schizophrenia Stigmatized?

1. Surgeon General's Report on Mental Health, chapter 1, http://www.surgeon general.gov/library/mentalhealth/chapter1/sec1.html#roots_stigma.

2. National Report Card on Health Care, http://www.cma.ca/multimedia/CMA /Content_Images/Inside_cma/Annual_Meeting/2008/GC_Bulletin/National _Report_Card_EN.pdf.

3. Harris/NAMI survey, http://www.nami.org/sstemplate.cfm?section =SchizophreniaSurvey.

4. E. B. Elbogen and S. C. Johnson (2009). The intricate link between violence and mental disorder. *Archives of General Psychiatry* 66:152–161. Quote on p. 157.

5. For evidence on this point, see R. Chase (2012). *The Physical Basis of Mental Illness*. Piscataway, NJ: Transaction.

6. Surgeon General's Report on Mental Health, chapter 1.

7. R. Descartes (1641, 1965). *Meditations*, no. IV. *A Discourse on Method and Other Works*. J. Epstein, ed. New York: Washington Square Press.

8. See the quotation from Hippocrates in chapter 12.

9. Only late in the twentieth century did investigative tools become sharp enough to detect the now obvious biomarkers.

10. B. Weiner (1995). *Judgments of Responsibility: A Foundation for a Theory of Social Conduct*. New York: Guilford Press.

11. C. Boorse (1975). On the distinction between disease and illness. *Philosophy and Public Affairs* 5:49–68.

12. B. G. Link et al. (1999). Public conceptions of mental illness: Labels, causes, dangerousness, and social distance. *American Journal of Public Health* 89: 1328–1333.

13. M. C. Angermeyer and H. Matschinger (1994). Lay beliefs about schizophrenic disorder: The results of a population survey in Germany. *Acta Psychiatrica Scandinavica* 89 (suppl. 382):39–45.

14. National Report Card on Health Care, http://www.cma.ca/multimedia /CMA/Content_Images/Inside_cma/Annual_Meeting/2008/GC_Bulletin/.

15. B. A. Pescosolido et al. (2010). "A disease like any other"? A decade of change in public reactions to schizophrenia, depression, and alcohol dependence. *American Journal of Psychiatry* 167:1321–1330. Quote on p. 1325.

Chapter 16. Just What Is Schizophrenia, Anyway?

1. M. S. Keshavan, H. A. Nasrallah, and R. Tandon (2011). Schizophrenia, "Just the facts" 6. Moving ahead with the schizophrenia concept: From the elephant to the mouse. *Schizophrenia Research* 127:3–13. Quote on p. 3.

2. A. Moskowitz and G. Heim (2011). Eugen Bleuler's *Dementia Praecox or the Group of Schizophrenias* (1911): A centenary appreciation and reconsideration. *Schizophrenia Bulletin* 37:471–479. Quote on p. 473.

3. *Diagnostic and Statistical Manual of Mental Disorders* (DSM), 5th ed. (2013). Arlington, VA: American Psychiatric Association.

4. R. E. Kendell et al. (1971). Diagnostic criteria of American and British psychiatrists. *Archives of General Psychiatry* 25:123–130.

5. The quote is on p. 129 of Kendell 1971.

6. Evidence of an association would be weakened by misdiagnoses based on subjective criteria, for example, if an individual carrying a true biomarker for schizophrenia were to be incorrectly diagnosed as having a different disorder or if an individual lacking any biomarker for schizophrenia were to be incorrectly diagnosed with schizophrenia.

7. E. M. Joyce and J. P. Roiser (2007). Cognitive heterogeneity in schizophrenia. *Current Opinion in Psychiatry* 20:268–272.

8. H. Bentsen et al. (2011). Bimodal distribution of polyunsaturated fatty acids in schizophrenia suggests two endophenotypes of the disorder. *Biological Psychiatry* 70:97–105.

9. C. Curtis et al. (2012). The genomic and transcriptomic architecture of 2,000 breast tumours reveals novel subgroups. *Nature* 486:346–352.

10. P. F. Sullivan et al. (2012). Family history of schizophrenia and bipolar disorder as risk factors for autism. *Archives of General Psychiatry* 69:1099–1103.

11. Cross-Disorder Group of the Psychiatric Genomics Consortium (2013). Identification of risk loci with shared effects on five major psychiatric disorders: a genome-wide analysis. *Lancet* 381:1371-1379. The "risk loci" identified in this study are variants of single DNA "letters," also known as single-nucleotide polymorphisms.

12. Keshavan, Nasrallah, and Tandon 2011. Quote on p.11.

13. M. J. Owen et al. (2011). Neurodevelopmental hypothesis of schizophrenia. *British Journal of Psychiatry* 198:173–175. Quote on p. 173.

14. S. E. Morris and T. R. Insel (2011). Reconceptualizing schizophrenia. *Schizophrenia Research* 127:1–2.

Chapter 18. When Did Schizophrenia First Appear, and Why Doesn't It Go Away?

1. A famous quotation from the distinguished American biologist, Theodosius Dobzhansky (1900–1975).

2. The technical term for reproductive success is *fitness.*

3. A detailed list of all the fertility studies is presented in M. C. Keller and G. Miller (2006). Resolving the paradox of common, harmful, heritable mental disorders: Which evolutionary genetic models work best? *Behavioral and Brain Sciences* 29:385–452.

4. The article by Keller and Miller (2006) contains a full airing of all the pertinent issues regarding schizophrenia. The main article is followed by 24 commentaries written by other experts in the field, with rebuttals by Keller and Miller. Together, the article and its commentaries provide a fine example of how scientists can argue about controversial topics without resorting to rhetorical devices unrelated to reason and facts.

5. The calculation is on p. 393 of Keller and Miller 2006. The authors assume that the negative effect of schizophrenia on fertility has remained unchanged from 1600 to the present.

6. Some evidence suggests that schizophrenia originated as recently as 1800 (as I discuss later in this chapter). If this hypothesis were to be proved, it would favor the idea that negative selection has not yet had time to eliminate all the risk-causing mutations.

7. D. F. Horrobin (2001). *The Madness of Adam and Eve: How Schizophrenia Shaped Humanity.* London: Bantam.

8. J. J. McGrath et al. (2004). A systematic review of the incidence of schizophrenia: The distribution of rates and the influence of sex, urbanicity, migrant status and methodology. *BMC Medicine* 2:13.

9. T. O'Reilly, R. Dunbar, and R. Bentall (2001). Schizotypy and creativity: An evolutionary connection? *Personality and Individual Differences* 31:1067–1078.

Some examples of persons with schizophrenia include Albert Einstein's son, Alan Alda's mother, Tennessee Williams's sister, and James Joyce's daughter.

10. D. Nettle and H. Clegg (2006). Schizotypy, creativity and mating success in humans. *Proceedings of the Royal Society B* 273:611–615. Although having sexual partners is not the same as having children, mating success is actually a better indicator of positive evolutionary selection than the number of offspring because the latter measure is confounded by condom use, family planning, and unreported children from extramarital affairs.

11. J. Haukka, J. Suvisaari, and J. Loönnqvist (2003). Fertility of patients with schizophrenia, their siblings, and the general population: A cohort study from 1950 to 1959 in Finland. *American Journal of Psychiatry* 160:460–463.

12. J. J. McGrath (2006). The romance of balancing selection versus the sober alternatives: Let the data rule. *Behavioral and Brain Sciences* 29:417–418.

13. A. Shaner, G. Miller, and J. Mintz (2004). Schizophrenia as one extreme of a sexually selected fitness indicator. *Schizophrenia Research* 70:101–109.

14. M. Lynch (2010). Rate, molecular spectrum, and consequences of human mutation. *Proceedings of the National Academy of Sciences USA* 107:961–968.

15. J. A. Tennessen et al. (2012). Evolution and functional impact of rare coding variation from deep sequencing of human exomes. *Science* 337:64–69. See also my discussion of rare mutations in chapter 4.

16. E. Hare (1988). Schizophrenia as a recent disease. *British Journal of Psychiatry* 153:521–531.

17. J. Haslam (1810, 1988). *Illustrations of Madness*. London: Routledge.

18. E. Shorter (1997). *A History of Psychiatry: From the Era of the Asylum to the Age of Prozac*. New York: John Wiley & Sons. Quote on p. 61.

19. Hare 1988. Quote on p. 525.

Chapter 19. Jim's Final Days (1998–1999)

1. J. R. Strawn, P. E. Keck Jr., and S. N. Caroff (2007). Neuroleptic malignant syndrome. *American Journal of Psychiatry* 16:870–876. Quotes on pp. 870 and 872.

Chapter 20. What Happens to People with Schizophrenia through the Years?

1. G. Harrison et al. (2001). Recovery from psychotic illness: A 15- and 25-year international follow-up study. *British Journal of Psychiatry* 178:506–517.

2. D. Novick et al. (2009). Recovery in the outpatient setting: 36-month results from the Schizophrenia Outpatients Health Outcomes (SOHO) study. *Schizophrenia Research* 108:223–230.

3. J. van Os and S. Kapur (2009). Schizophrenia. *Lancet* 374:635–645.

4. M. Bertelsen et al. (2008). Five-year follow-up of a randomized multicenter trial of intensive early intervention vs. standard treatment for patients with a first episode of psychotic illness. *Archives of General Psychiatry* 65:762–771.

5. D. Novick et al. (2010). Predictors and clinical consequences of non-adherence with antipsychotic medication in the outpatient treatment of schizophrenia. *Psychiatry Research* 176:109–113.

6. Exceptionally, drugs can be administered without the patient's permission in rare, legally mandated cases.

7. J. McGrath et al. (2008). Schizophrenia: A concise overview of incidence, prevalence, and mortality. *Epidemiologic Reviews* 30:67–76.

Chapter 21. Reflections

1. For elaboration of these arguments, see R. Chase (2012). *The Physical Basis of Mental Illness*. Piscataway, NJ: Transaction.

Epilogue

1. My own career followed a similar path. I studied psychology as a university undergraduate, but later enrolled in a graduate program focused on neuroscience. Driven as I was by my brother's illness, I might have looked to psychoanalysis as a career option if my education had come a decade earlier, but the field of neuroscience had already begun to bloom by 1965, and I could not resist its attractions.

2. S. Saha et al. (2005). A systematic review of the prevalence of schizophrenia. *Public Library of Science Medicine* 2(5):e141.

3. Editorial (2010). A decade for psychiatric disorders. *Nature* 463:9.

4. T. R. Insel (2012). Next-generation treatments for mental disorders. *Science Translational Medicine* 4: 155ps19.

5. S. L. Clark, D. E. Adkins, and E. J. C. G. van den Oord (2011). Analysis of efficacy and side effects in CATIE demonstrates drug response subgroups and potential for personalized medicine. *Schizophrenia Research* 132:114–120.

Glossary

action potential. A pulselike electrical event during which current flows briefly inward and then outward across the neuronal membrane. The action potential is the only electrical signal that travels over long distances in the nervous system. It is conducted along *axons*; when it reaches the end of the axon, it triggers the release of one or more *neurotransmitter substances*.

affect. Subjective feelings or expressed emotions, such as joy, sadness, anger, and fear.

allele. One of two or more alternative forms of a *gene*. Alternative forms arise from mutations; they sometimes produce a variation in the heritable characteristic that is coded for by the gene. Each gene is represented by two alleles, one on each of the paired chromosomes. Also known as a *gene variant*.

antagonist (pharmacological). A drug that blocks the effects of another drug or natural body chemical, for example, a drug that blocks a *neurotransmitter*.

axon. The extended processes of nerve cells that function to transmit action potentials over distances ranging from a few hundred micrometers to a meter or more. Each axon is covered with a fatty substance, myelin, that serves as an electrical insulator.

biomarker. Generally, a biological feature that provides information on the status of a system. Biomarkers for schizophrenia may be genetic, neuroanatomical, biochemical, or physiological. They can provide clues to mechanisms responsible for the disease, but only if they can be shown to be causes, not consequences of the disease.

cognition. Unobservable mental activities that underlie the acquisition and processing of knowledge. Includes sensory perception, attention, memory, planning, use of language, and reasoning.

concordance. A measure used in twin studies to determine the extent to which a disease is inherited. Investigators first locate one twin with the disease, say schizophrenia. If they find that the other twin has the same disease, the pair is said to be concordant for that disease.

cortex. Brain tissue that is characterized by a layered arrangement of nerve cells. The single word "cortex" is often used in reference to the cerebral cortex, which covers nearly the entire surface of the brain and serves numerous high-level functions. However, other brain structures, such as the *hippocampus*, also have cortical architectures.

delusion. A belief in something that has no basis in reality. Many people with schizophrenia believe that they are Jesus Christ.

dementia praecox. Latin for premature dementia or early insanity. The original name for the disorder that is now known as schizophrenia.

dendrite. Slender, multibranched extensions of neurons. Their function is to receive messages from other neurons, which are transmitted across synapses. Neurons typically have thousands of synaptic sites on their dendrites, sometimes hundreds of thousands.

disorganized behavior. A so-called *positive symptom* in schizophrenia. Examples include inappropriate gestures, inappropriate emotional expressions, seemingly random or repetitive movements, and impulsivity.

disorganized speech. A so-called *positive symptom* in schizophrenia. Typically involves jumbling together of words and phrases in an incoherent manner.

DNA. Abbreviation for the large molecule, deoxyribonucleic acid, which has the structure of a double helix. It is essentially a long chain of smaller molecules, called nucleotides, which occur as four types, or "letters." All the information that we inherit from our parents is contained in the precise order of nucleotides. See also *RNA*.

dualism. The philosophy of mind that assumes that mind is a thing separate from, and independent of, the brain. Often associated with the writings of René Descartes (1596–1650). In contrast to *monism*.

environment. For epidemiologists and geneticists, the environment means everything that a person is exposed to outside of himself or herself. It includes physical, social, and cultural aspects. All human traits result from an interaction between genes and the environment.

epidemiology. The study of the distributions and patterns of medically related conditions in defined human populations. Epidemiologists use statistical methods to help identify causes and risk factors for diseases.

epigenetics. The study of heritable changes in traits caused by mechanisms other than changes in *DNA*. The best known of these mechanisms involves modifications to the proteins that surround the *DNA* and that regulate the read-out (transcription) of its genes.

executive control functions. A loosely defined set of skills and processes that together govern the organization of behavior. Examples include attention, short-term memory, planning, problem solving, and the initiation of actions. The neural control of these functions resides mostly in the prefrontal cortex.

gene. The fundamental physical unit of heredity. In molecular terms, a gene comprises a segment of *DNA*. When the gene is activated (transcribed), it is copied into *RNA*, which then directs the synthesis of a protein. Hence, each gene typically codes for, and makes, a single protein.

genetics. The study of biological heredity, especially the mechanisms of inheritance and the variation in traits among individuals and species. Largely concerned with genes.

gene variant. Synonym for *allele*.

genome. All the inherited information that is contained within an individual's DNA.

hallucination. A subjective experience in which a person perceives something that is not actually there. Although hallucinations can occur in any sensory modality, auditory hallucinations are most common in schizophrenia, for example, when a patient hears her father speaking to her although her father is not present.

heritability. In scientific usage, referring to the proportion of variation in a particular trait that is due to variation in the genes responsible for that trait. It does *not* describe the extent to which the trait is caused by genetic influences, nor can it be applied to individuals. Heritability is calculated for a defined population at a defined time.

hippocampus. Located near the center of the brain (on both right and left sides), the hippocampus is a distinctive neural structure that plays an important role in forming memories for events and the contexts in which they occur.

incidence. The number of *new* cases of a disease in one year divided by the number of people in the population.

interneuron. A *neuron* type that is neither a sensory neuron nor a motor neuron. Interneurons are small. When active, they usually inhibit the activity of other neurons through *synapses*.

microcircuit. Small networks containing several hundred or a few thousand nerve cells that are connected with one another through synapses. Microcircuits of a particular design are found throughout the cerebral *cortex*. They constitute the basic "computing" units responsible for many cognitive functions.

monism. The philosophy that assumes that only physical things exist and that mind is a subjective phenomenon that arises from physiological activity in the brain. In contrast to *dualism*.

mutation. A change in the *DNA* sequence that constitutes a *gene*. A mutation may, or may not, produce a variation in an observable trait.

negative symptoms. Attributes that are weakened or absent in people with schizophrenia. Examples include poverty of thought, reduced affect, reduced ambition, and few social interactions.

neurodevelopment. The process of forming the brain and its associated nervous system from information contained in the genome. Begins in the embryo and continues through to about age 30.

neuron (nerve cell). An electrically excitable cell that integrates and transmits information in the nervous system. Its principal parts are the cell body (soma), *axon*, and *dendrites*. There are many distinct types of neurons, each distinguished by anatomical form, electrical signaling properties, neurochemistry, and connections within the nervous system.

neuropeptide. Peptides are biological compounds containing two or more amino acids; thus, they are like proteins, but smaller. Many different neuropeptides function either as conventional *neurotransmitters* or as modulators of neuronal activity.

neuroscience. The study of all aspects of nerve cells, from the physics of light sensation to the chemistry of pain, from the shapes of synapses to the correlates of consciousness. The Society for Neuroscience, an organization of researchers based primarily in the United States, has more than 40,000 members.

neurotransmitter. A chemical substance released by one nerve cell to influence the physiological activity of another nerve cell. Neurotransmitters are usually released at *synapses*. Some are inhibitory, some excitatory, and some have complex metabolic effects. About 100 different molecules serve as neurotransmitters.

neurotransmitter receptor. A type of molecule that resides within the cell membrane of nerve cells. It functions to bind (capture) neurotransmitters and mediate their effects. While an individual receptor binds just one specific type of neurotransmitter, a single neurotransmitter may be bound by many different receptor types, each of which initiates a unique physiological effect.

paranoia. A particular kind of *delusion*. Most commonly in schizophrenia, the patient has the irrational belief that he or she is the target of a plot, is being pursued, or is otherwise oppressed (persecutory paranoia). Less commonly, the patient believes that he or she is someone very important or famous (grandiose paranoia).

positive symptoms. Psychological phenomena and behaviors found in people with schizophrenia but not ordinarily found in healthy individuals. Mainly hallucinations, delusions, incoherent speech, disorganized thought, and disorganized behavior.

prefrontal cortex. The cortical area at the extreme anterior tip of the frontal lobe. It is important for short-term ("working") memory and *executive control functions*. Damage to this area causes apathy, poor judgment, and the inability to plan actions. The prefrontal cortex is much larger in humans than in nonhuman species.

prevalence. Expressed as a percentage, or rate, it is the number of people who have a disease divided by the total number of people in the population. Several different rates can be estimated depending on the period of time covered, for example, a particular year or a particular day. The lifetime prevalence is the proportion of individuals in the population who have ever manifested the disease and who are alive on a given day. The lifetime morbid risk is a theoretical measure that encompasses the entire lifetime both past and future and includes those deceased at the time of the survey.

prospective/retrospective studies. Two types of epidemiologic and psychiatric investigations, both of which seek to identify causes and risk factors for diseases. Prospective studies select individuals for inclusion in the study before any of them have shown signs of disease. Retrospective studies find affected individuals in hospital records or other documentary sources; relevant data concerning these cases are then compared with data from a matched group of healthy individuals.

protein. A type of large biological molecule. Proteins build body structures, participate in metabolic processes, support cell-to-cell communications, and perform a variety of other functions. The "central dogma" of molecular biology states that *DNA* makes *RNA* makes protein. Thus, each gene carries the DNA code for making a particular protein.

psychiatry. The medical specialty that deals with mental illnesses. Doctors who work in this field are called psychiatrists.

psychoanalysis. A particular type of *psychotherapy* derived from the ideas of Sigmund Freud. A psychoanalyst is someone who treats patients using psychoanalysis.

psychosis. The state of mind in which thinking becomes irrational or severely disturbed. Psychotic individuals are said to lose contact with reality due to *delusions* or *hallucinations*. The most common psychotic diseases are schizophrenia and bipolar disorder.

psychotherapy. A therapy that engages the patient in talking. A person who administers psychotherapy, whether a psychiatrist or a nonmedical professional, is known as a psychotherapist.

RNA. Abbreviation for the large molecule, ribonucleic acid. Like *DNA*, it is composed of four different nucleotides. RNA is made from *DNA* using special enzymes in a process called transcription. There are several types of RNA, each with related but different functions in processing genetic information. One important function is to build proteins from amino acids.

stigma. In earlier times, a stigma was a distinguishing mark on the skin. Today, it is the social disgrace carried by people who have certain diseases or life circumstances or other factors that set them apart in a perceived negative way.

synapse. Anatomically, it is a tiny, specialized region of the neuronal membrane that can only be seen with an electron microscope. Physiologically, it is the site at which one *neuron* communicates with another. Synaptic transmission occurs when a *neurotransmitter* is released from one neuron's *axon*, diffuses across a very narrow gap, and is bound by a receptor on the other neuron's *dendrite*.

temporal lobe. One of the four major subdivisions of the cerebral *cortex*, it occupies the lower region on each side of the brain. Its functions include high-level visual and auditory processing, speech production, and speech comprehension.

Suggested Readings

Chase, Ronald. *The Physical Basis of Mental Illness*. Piscataway, NJ: Transaction, 2012.

In my earlier book, I explain how a person's philosophical assumptions about the mind influence his or her attitudes toward mental illness. I argue that mental illness is in the brain, not in the mind.

Collins, Francis. *The Language of Life: DNA and the Revolution in Personalized Medicine*. New York: Harper, 2010.

The author was a leading investigator in the first complete description of the human genome; he later became head of the U.S. National Institutes of Health. In this popular work, he describes the science of molecular biology in readily understandable terms and outlines the prospects for its application in medicine. Gushes with optimism.

Gottesman, Irving I. *Schizophrenia Genesis: The Origins of Madness*. New York: W. H. Freeman, 1991.

This book draws attention to the importance of family studies, twin studies, and adoption studies. Although somewhat dated in its treatment of other topics, its clarity and its inclusion of first-person "anguished accounts" make it a valuable read.

Healy, David. *The Creation of Psychopharmacology*. Cambridge, MA: Harvard University Press, 2002.

The author tells the fascinating stories of how psychiatric drugs, especially antipsychotic drugs, were discovered, developed, and marketed. In many cases, the drugs were discovered by accident, rather than by design or scientific experimentation. The controlling influences of the pharmaceutical industry are highlighted.

Hinshaw, Stephen P. *The Mark of Shame: Stigma of Mental Illness and an Agenda for Change*. New York: Oxford University Press, 2009.

In addition to a comprehensive analysis of stigma from historical, psychological, sociological, and evolutionary perspectives, this book includes a full discussion of what can be done about it.

LeDoux, Joseph. *Synaptic Self: How Our Brains Become Who We Are*. New York: Penguin, 2003.

Although only part of the book deals specifically with mental illness, as a whole it provides an excellent, highly readable introduction to neuroscience. The main features of human subjective experience are shown to derive more from what occurs at tiny synapses than from the levels of brain chemicals.

Mueser, Kim T., and Gingerich, Susan. *The Complete Family Guide to Schizophrenia: Helping Your Loved One Get the Most Out of Life*. New York: Guilford, 2006.

This is a detailed guide to navigating the problems encountered by families that must deal with schizophrenia. It offers both practical and psychological advice.

Nettle, Daniel. *Strong Imagination: Madness, Creativity and Human Nature*. New York: Oxford University Press, 2001.

The contention is that schizophrenia evolved and persists because it is linked to creativity. The author engages us by building his argument from diverse scientific, cultural, and artistic sources. Read the book as a good example of evolutionary speculation but remain skeptical about the main hypothesis.

Rose, Hilary, and Rose, Steven. *Genes, Cells and Brains: The Promethean Promises of the New Biology*. London: Verso, 2013.

In this radical critique of neuroscience, gene technology, and molecular biology, the authors highlight the disappointing results, particularly with respect to clinical benefits. The book is useful as a counterpoint to the exuberant claims made by Francis Collins in the book listed above. It tells us that the payoffs of research may arrive later than most of us expect.

Shorter, Edward. *A History of Psychiatry: From the Era of the Asylum to the Age of Prozac*. New York: John Wiley & Sons, 1997.

This highly readable account weaves a rich tapestry of facts interlaced with the author's forthright opinions. Schizophrenia appears as just one of many related human conditions for which physicians have sought effective treatments.

Torrey, E. Fuller. *Surviving Schizophrenia: A Manual for Families, Consumers, and Providers*. New York: Harper, 2006 (5th edition).

The author, a psychiatrist, has written many influential books about schizophrenia. This accessible volume is a comprehensive compendium of facts mixed with the author's sometimes quirky opinions. It summarizes medical and scientific knowledge, offers a variety of practical advice, and discusses public policy issues. At 576 pages in length, it is not a quick read.

United States Department of Health and Human Services together with other
U.S. government agencies, *Schizophrenia: Causes, Symptoms, Signs, Diagnosis
and Treatments*. CreateSpace (a subsidiary of Amazon.com), 2012.
A very brief summary (48 pages) of essential information for persons developing schizophrenia, their family members, and friends.

Index